I0084672

HAVE YOU PLANNED YOUR
HEART ATTACK?

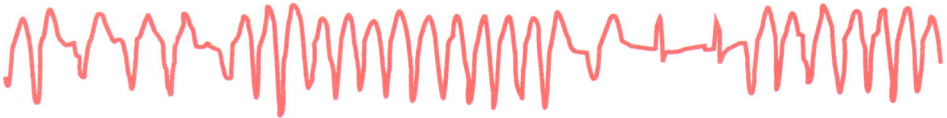

DR WARRICK BISHOP

WHAT YOU NEED TO KNOW
TO UNDERSTAND AND
REDUCE YOUR RISK

a discussion for patients and doctors

HAVE YOU PLANNED YOUR HEART ATTACK?

WHAT YOU NEED TO KNOW TO UNDERSTAND AND REDUCE YOUR RISK

bringing the future into the present

This book is for you, if you:

- want to reduce your risk of a heart attack;
- have high cholesterol and are not sure about taking statins;
- suffer side-effects from statins;
- come from a family with 'bad' hearts;
- just want to know what's going on with your heart;
- want to know more about cardiac CT imaging;
- would enjoy an informative read about the main killer of our generation;
- believe prevention is better than cure, or
- are a doctor wanting more information about risk or need a book you can recommend to your patients.

This book is also for you, if you have a heart.

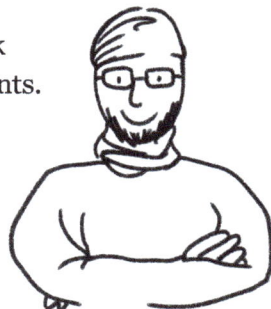

Publisher's Note

The author and editors of this publication have made every effort to provide information that is accurate and complete as of the date of publication. Readers are advised not to rely on the information provided without consulting their own medical advisers. It is the responsibility of the reader's treating physician or specialist, who relies on experience and knowledge about the patient, to determine the condition of, and the best treatment for, the reader. The information contained in this publication is provided without warranty of any kind. The author and editors disclaim responsibility for any errors, mis-statements, typographical errors or omissions in this publication.

© 2016 Warrick Bishop MB BS FRACP

This publication is copyright. Other than for the purposes of and subject to the conditions prescribed under the Copyright Act, no part of it may in any form or by any means (electronic, mechanical, micro-copying, photocopying, recording or otherwise) be reproduced, stored in a retrieval system or transmitted without prior written permission.

Any information reproduced herein which has been obtained from any other copyright owner has been reproduced with that copyright owner's permission but does not purport to be an accurate reproduction. Inquiries should be addressed to the publishers.

National Library of Australia Cataloguing-in-Publication entry

Author:	Bishop, Dr Warrick
Title:	Have You Planned Your Heart Attack?
POD ISBN:	978-0-646-96267-2
Subject:	Cardiac health care

Published:	Dr Warrick Bishop
Ghost written:	Penelope Edman
Cover design:	Doodlefish Web Design
Internal design:	Cathy McAuliffe Design
Illustrations:	Cathy McAuliffe Design
Printed on Demand:	Ingram Spark

To my parents, Chris and Marie,
who taught me persistence, quality,
integrity and humility the best way
possible - by example.

Contents

Foreword

If you're reading this, you can reasonably assume, despite my journalistic lifestyle and my cholesterol level, that I am still alive. My cardiologist, who is the author and publisher of this book, would not have prefaced a work on cardiac health with the thoughts of a dead patient. So I'm still here. That's the good news. Thanks, Doc!

The bad news is, that in Australia, heart failure is the cause of more than 30 percent of deaths every year and most of these are due to coronary heart disease. This book confronts that stark reality in a readable, informative and practical way.

Are we, by diet and lifestyle, our own worst enemies? Or are we hapless victims of a cruelly indifferent genetic lottery? And the harder question: in either of those alternatives, what can we do about it?

In my work as a journalist I travel to some of the most remote parts of the world and it slowly occurred to me that Afghanistan or Antarctica would be inconvenient spots to suffer a heart attack. As you will learn from this book, the traditional medical evaluations of the state of the heart are often just highly educated guess work. Cardiologists admit you can pass a stress test one week and die the next. Because I needed to get to the heart of the matter, I wanted to know what was going on in there.

Your author, and my cardiologist, Warrick Bishop, is a lean and determined-looking man whose shaven head and athletic fitness bring to mind Vladimir Putin, without the unhappy associations. Indeed, what drew me to Dr Bishop was that he specialises in looking inside the working heart.

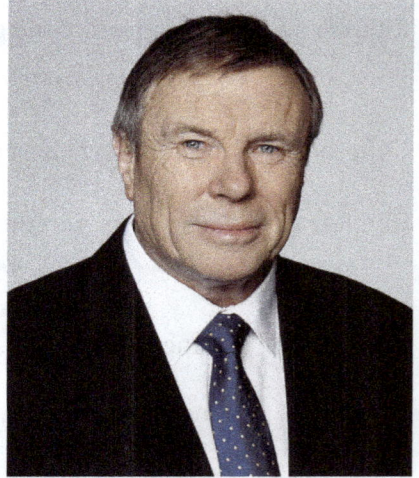

Using non-invasive imaging technology, he sees inside our coronary arteries to determine just how rusted and encrusted the pipes have become.

For you and me, Warrick Bishop's picture is worth a thousand words.

It's our hearts, the very lifeblood of our earthly existence, he is speaking about in his consulting room and writing about here. In a world of conflicting expert opinion, of contradictory scientific surveys, of fads and fancies and fierce dietary debate, Warrick Bishop is leading us towards some diagnostic certainty. If we know what's actually happening inside, then we have a basis for remedial action.

In my case Warrick Bishop tells me that if I lay off the carbs and keep the cholesterol down, I should get an extra couple of years in the Eventide Home. Maybe, eventually, I'll see you there. In the meantime, enjoy the book.

CHARLES WOOLEY

Hobart-based international television journalist and author

Hobart, Tasmania, Australia

February 2016

Preface

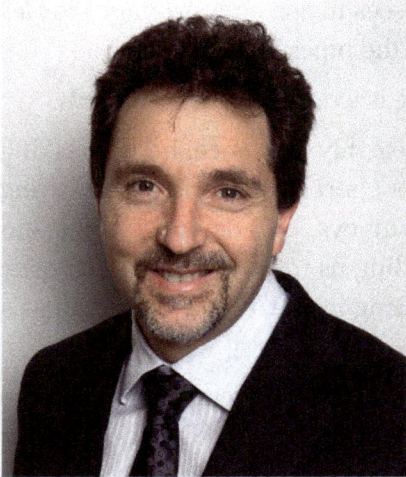

Dr Warrick Bishop, I applaud you in writing this book. You cover an extremely important topic as one in two people will have coronary vascular disease and one in three will die from it.

The deficiencies of currently endorsed risk evaluation strategies are well known – risk can be under-predicted by up to 57 percent in high-risk groups and over-predicted by up to 287 percent in low-risk groups.

You clearly identify the Holy Grail of coronary vascular disease, predicting which plaques are likely to rupture, and doing everything you can to prevent that without resorting to blanket therapy. That a patient-centric approach is needed is clear and I share your vision that cardiac CT is the way this will be achieved. You are not a lone voice in this; indeed, there are many who share your enthusiasm for what the technology has to offer.

Challenging time-honoured approaches will always draw criticism as there is inherent inertia to change. Most people do today what they did yesterday which, in the terms of most cardiologists, is consultation and functional testing.

We as clinicians cannot simply continue unthinkingly, allowing the high residual burden of risk to keep claiming our patients' livelihoods and lives.

As with many revolutions, there will need to be a phase of evaluation and a groundswell of support before wholesale adoption. We sit on this threshold right now and I am confident, that within a few years, there will be publications vindicating the practice you, I and others have advocated over the past 10 years.

You have produced a very informative work that is entertaining to read. You are to be congratulated in guiding patients and doctors alike through the complexities of coronary artery disease. I will certainly recommend this book to patients and colleagues.

DANIEL FRIEDMAN

Consultant, imaging and interventional cardiologist

Prince of Wales Private and Public Hospitals
Sydney, New South Wales, Australia

June 2016

Dr Daniel Friedman has been involved in Cardiac CTA since its inception and is an acknowledged leader in the field of Cardiac CT in Australia. He held the inaugural Chair of the ANZ International Regional Committee of the (American) Society of Cardiovascular CT and is a founding member of the ANZ CTCA Conjoint Committee. He is the Founder and Director of the Australian Institute of Cardiovascular CT which runs advanced cardiac CT training programs for cardiologists, radiologists and nuclear medicine physicians. He is the imaging editor for the peer-reviewed Australian cardiac journal Heart, Lung and Circulation.

上医医未病之病
中医医将病之病
下医医已病之病
～黄帝：内経～

Superior doctors prevent the disease.
Mediocre doctors treat the disease before evident.
Inferior doctors treat the full-blown disease.

HAUG DEE: NAI-CHING

2600BC

first Chinese medical text

Introduction -
Not good enough!

On a Saturday in May of 2005, a 52-year-old man collapsed, having had a cardiac arrest during a fun run. I noticed the commotion as I was driving past on my way to work and stopped. Several other runners, including a general practitioner, had already stopped to help and the Ambulance Service was in attendance. I am pleased to report that, with everyone's input, the man was resuscitated, taken to hospital and received stenting to the main artery down the front of his heart. The outcome was so good that it later made the front page of the local newspaper.

When I arrived at work on the Monday I felt fairly pleased to have been a contributor to such a positive outcome. Before I could become too proud, however, one of my staff pointed out that I had seen the very same gentleman two years earlier for an exercise treadmill test. The test had been normal and I had reassured him that "everything's okay". This revelation shocked me! Had I done the wrong thing by this man? Had I misinterpreted the test? Were there other factors of which I had not been aware? As it turned out, I had done nothing wrong; the test was appropriately reported and he was given reassurance consistent with his risk assessment at that time. In fact, I had suggested he start low-dose aspirin because of his history of mildly elevated blood pressure, for which he was on treatment.

Not good enough!

My original assessment in 2003 had limitations. This book is about how, with today's technology, we can do better – potentially much better. It is about improved dealing with risk through investigation and management. I do not wish, ever, to be in a situation again when I reassure a patient and then find that person has suffered a heart attack, let alone be involved in that person's resuscitation! That man's collapse was over 10 years ago and technology has changed so that we can deal with these situations in a different way.

ACCORDING TO THE HEART FOUNDATION, ABOUT 55,000 AUSTRALIANS SUFFER A HEART ATTACK EACH YEAR.

According to the Heart Foundation, about 55,000 Australians suffer a heart attack each year. This equates to one heart attack every 10 minutes.

'Heart attack' is a layman's term referring to a narrowing or blockage of the coronary arteries that can kill, or requires some form of medical intervention such as medication, time in a hospital, balloons or stents, or coronary artery bypass grafting.

As a cardiologist, I have not yet met a patient who expected to have a problem; patients do not put into their diaries "possible problem with my heart next week". **Yet, what if we could be forewarned about, or prepared for, a potential problem with our coronary arteries?**

What if we were able to put in place preventative measures that may avert a problem? What if we were able to take away the surprise of a heart attack occurring 'out of the blue' and replace possible fear with prepared understanding?

....

What if we could PLAN NOT to have a heart attack?

....

Primary prevention …

PETER was a 35-year-old male with high cholesterol who had tried cholesterol-lowering tablets but had suffered aches and pains. He really didn't want to be on medication unless it was clearly indicated. At our first meeting, he was fit and well, and was not on any regular medication. There was no history of premature coronary artery disease in his family although both his parents had had elevated cholesterol. His lipid profile was:

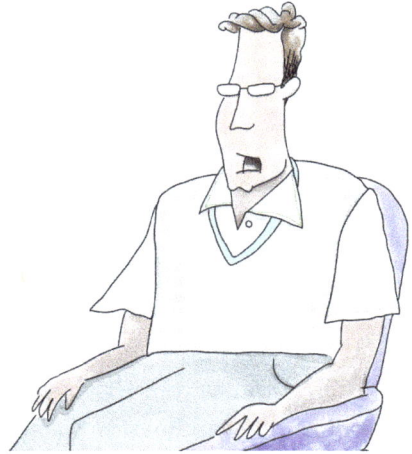

Total Cholesterol (TC)	11.0	ideally < (less than) 5.0 mmol/l
Triglycerides (TG)	1.9	ideally <2.0 mmol/l
High Density Lipoprotein (HDL)	1.0	ideally > (greater than) 1.0 mmol/l
TC to HDL ratio	11.0	ideally <4.0 ratio
Non HDL	10.0	ideally <4.0 mmol/l
Low Density Lipoprotein (LDL)	9.1	ideally <2.5 mmol/l

These levels of cholesterol are high and concerning. The Australian absolute cardiovascular disease risk calculator estimated Peter's risk at greater than 15 percent chance of an event in the next five years or over 30 percent in 10 years. This was a very high risk.

We spoke at some length about the role of scanning his heart to provide more information about the state of his arteries, in a bid to determine in more detail what his risk might be. I explained that he was younger than usual for such scanning. I also explained the risk of x-ray exposure and of possible contrast reactions.

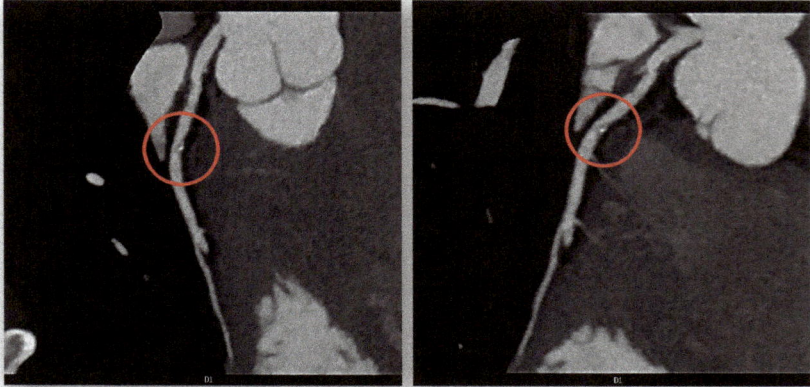

Peter was keen to undergo scanning so that he could be as well informed as possible and so make the best decisions for his care. He was married with three children and he didn't want to leave his heart health to chance. Above are the images we obtained.

The calcium score was three and this would generally suggest a low risk of an event over the next 5 to 10 years. However, as can be seen from the images above, there is a significant amount of non-calcific plaque which carries a high risk of an event over the next 5 to 10 years if left unattended.

I will explain plaque and other terminology soon.

This information was what Peter needed to know to be clear about his health management. I indicated that he would benefit from treatment. The pictures were explicit and gone were his doubts about the benefits of taking medication.

He is now on aspirin and two cholesterol-lowering medications, and has also embraced significant lifestyle changes. The result is a major turn-around in the management of his cardiovascular risk. He is happy with the outcome and is positive about being informed and proactive.

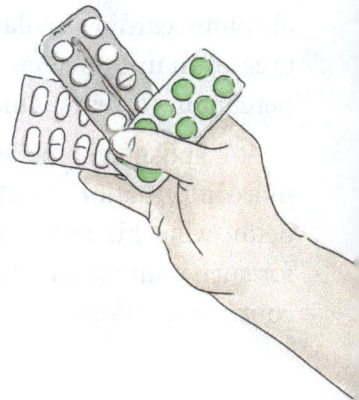

This is primary preventative cardiology – or much earlier intervention than traditionally undertaken – and is the fundamental focus of this book.

Treatment …

Historically, the detection and the treatment of coronary artery disease have been related to either the presence of symptoms or the occurrence of an event, such as a heart attack. Once a patient has been diagnosed as having coronary heart disease, the way forward is very clear: re-establish or improve the blood flow and put in place secondary prevention strategies to reduce the risk of a recurrence. Methods used to reduce recurrence include use of medication, reducing cholesterol levels and lifestyle modifications.

The situation is not as clear-cut, however, when it involves patients who have not had a problem. They do not display any symptoms nor have they been defined as having a problem. Yet, they might be at high risk because of indicators such as cholesterol levels or high blood pressure or diabetes or even smoking.

The treatment for that risk, prior to an event, is *primary prevention* – and this is where our interest lies. The difficulty with primary prevention is that it involves **treatment of the unknown.**

Although important in its own right, secondary prevention of coronary artery disease, that treatment which happens after diagnosis, will not receive much attention in this book. The data around secondary prevention is very clear and I do not believe there is any need for an alternative interpretation. Its significance for me wearing my 'preventative cardiology' hat is, however, that secondary prevention is late, in fact potentially **too late,** in the process.

Let's avoid the first event …

My objective in this book is to explore how to *avoid the first event.* When coronary artery disease is diagnosed at the time of the event, the time the patient has chest pain or shortness of breath or a major adverse coronary event, the patient has already developed a 'disease'. For me, to ***prevent*** chest pain or heart attack in the first place, to prevent the development of 'disease', is the Holy Grail of preventative cardiology.

Current primary prevention practice is based on *risk assessments*. I believe this has scope for re-evaluation.

The way we evaluate and calculate risk in individuals is based on **observational data.** This means that, over the years, databases have been compiled of features and factors found in individuals who have had coronary artery disease. The occurrence of those features and factors then lends weight to their being used as predictors for people before they have an event. Observational data collected from a large number of patients who have had heart attacks indicate that factors such as:

- increasing age;
- being male;
- cholesterol levels;
- increased blood pressure;
- diabetic status, and
- smoking

all feature as **associations** of having a possible a coronary event.   The important thing is that these associations are not necessarily what has **caused** the problem. This means that there can be people who are high-risk based on such factors, yet they will not have an event.

Understanding that our risk evaluation is based on associations and not causations is central to the following discussion.

Another significant factor is that today's CT imaging of the heart offers us an ability to evaluate the health of an individual's arteries **before** the onset of a problem. **This is a paradigm shift in the conventional management of coronary artery disease.** Yet, although cardiac CT imaging has been generally available for the past five to 10 years, it has not yet been broadly taken up.

An exploration of the exciting opportunities that cardiac imaging offers is also crucial to this book.

Although formalised guidelines or recommendations do not exist for some of the issues I will cover, I plan to use a logical and systematic approach, based on science that is available today, to discuss the case for a much broader understanding and application of preventative cardiology. Based on this information, I extend a two-fold invitation:

- **to patients,** to engage their doctors in a meaningful discussion about their heart health and well-being, and

- **to doctors,** to look into these issues with an open mind, with the best patient outcome as a priority.

It is a win-win situation for everyone.

page 15 credit: The Mercury *(News Ltd), Tuesday 17 May 2005, page 1; used with permission*

Let's explore …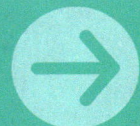

The argument for a re-evaluation of our approach to primary prevention in cardiac health care management

As a GP, I have been referring patients to Dr Bishop for around 10 years now. When speaking with me later, patients who have seen Dr Bishop highlight his communication skills and say that he explains their cardiac conditions to them in such a way that they can easily understand and, therefore, they feel comfortable with their treatment. His approachable, down-to-earth manner makes patients feel respected and at ease.

Deborah Peters, GP, Hobart

Chapter 1 -
Understanding your heart

IN THIS CHAPTER WE LOOK AT 👁

> the heart structure and its vulnerability

> symptoms and heart attack

No-one needs to be convinced about the importance of the heart for a healthy, well-functioning body. We all know that the heart is one of the critical organs necessary to sustain life.

The heart is a large muscle that pumps blood through our bodies to supply nutrients and oxygen, and also to remove waste such as carbon dioxide. It can be likened to a car engine, with compression chambers and valves, an electrical system and a set of fuel lines. Critical to the heart's operation are three major arteries, the coronary arteries. These are the fuel lines which carry blood to the heart muscle so that it can contract rhythmically, pumping blood to the body, 35 million times every year. As in a car engine, these lines can become blocked. This is the problem which concerns us.

CARDIOVASCULAR DISEASE involves heart and blood vessel diseases and includes stroke.

It affects one in six Australians, or 3.7 million people, and kills one Australian every 12 minutes.

Cardiovascular disease is often the main cause of hospitalisations in a given year.

We all know people who have had heart problems and it is very likely that someone close to us, either family or friend, has suffered a heart attack or died after one. Although 'heart attack' is not a medical term, it is commonly used to refer to a major heart-related event that can end life or put the person in hospital. Such an event is most commonly associated with a full, or near-complete, occlusion, or blockage, of a coronary artery (one of the 'fuel lines') and the subsequent consequences.

Dealing with such events has focussed on the two-fold treatment of the consequences: firstly, understanding where the problem is so that improved blood flow can be re-established and secondly, trying to prevent recurrences. The way

23

forward is clear: improve the blood flow and put in place preventative strategies to reduce the risk of any repeat events [1-3].

However, I believe there is another step which is often overlooked because the scientific evidence to support it is not as strong as for the above-mentioned best attempts to prevent the second heart attack. The issue around attempting to prevent problems **before** they manifest themselves with serious or fatal consequences is that the supporting data around the early detection of potential trouble is often anecdotal and not well supported by evidence-based trials and literature [4-7]. When trying to stave off repeat events, there are few such issues. A major cardiac event, an obvious problem, has occurred.

It is my contention that treatment can be instigated *before* clear indicators of a cardiac event are so obvious.

Typically, individual risk is evaluated using **associations** demonstrated in **population** studies. Yet, this presents inherent problems as the risk may be *low for the population* but it is ***100 percent** for the individual* who has the event!

***Symptoms* that point to *potential* problems in the coronary artery system are:**

- angina, or chest pain on exertion;
- shortness of breath on exertion, and
- acute coronary syndrome, manifested by chest pain at rest, leading to damage or death of part of the heart.

These are caused by:

- the build-up of plaque in the artery which
- leads to a narrowing of the vessel through which the blood is being pumped.

***Plaque*, the build-up of cholesterol, scavenger cells, scar tissue and calcium in the wall of the artery which is generally very localised, can be linked to a variety of *associations*, including:**

- age;
- sex;

- smoking;
- cholesterol level;
- high blood pressure, and/or
- diabetes

which can combine to influence the development of coronary artery disease.

This early, or **primary,** prevention which I am advocating attempts to prevent the development of coronary disease in a patient who has not suffered an event but indicators suggest could be at risk.

Before discussing more precise evaluation for primary prevention, we need to look at some basics.

Groundwork: the heart

Let's return to the analogy of our car engine.

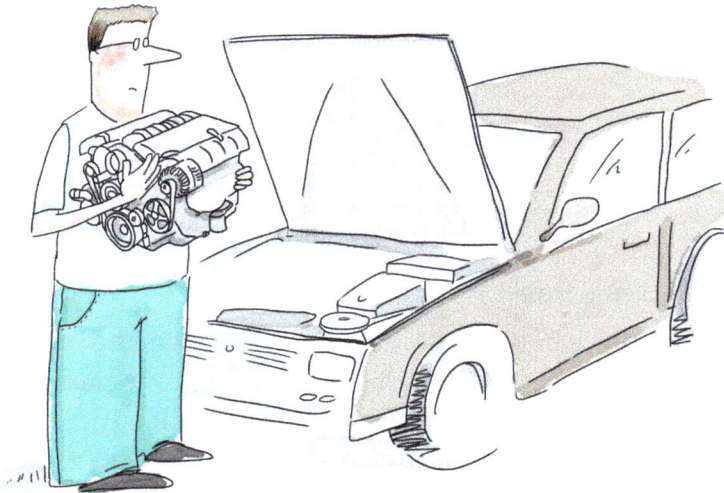

As a car engine has an **electrical system** for timing, so does the heart. The electrical system in the heart ensures synchronicity and coordinated contraction throughout the heart. It also allows a mechanism for acceleration and deceleration.

A car has **pistons** and **valves.** This is the engine block, the part that generates the power. So, within the heart, the pistons are the compression chambers, the main one being the **ventricle,** and the valves which stop the blood flowing back from where it came.

The car engine also requires a **fuel line** to supply the engine block. In the human heart, the fuel lines are the **coronary arteries** that literally provide the life blood to the engine block, the muscle that is the heart.

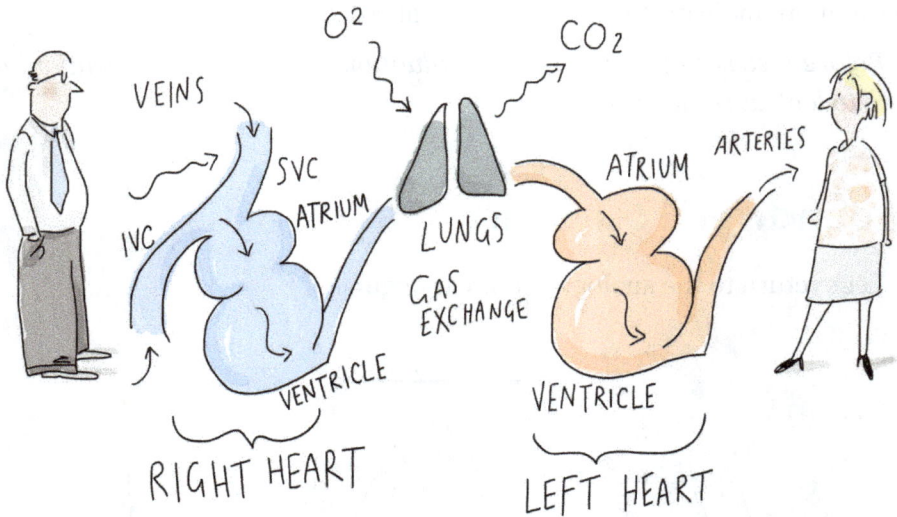

A schematic showing the flow of the blood through the heart from the veins to the arteries.

The heart is a four-chambered structure.

There are two chambers on the right-hand side and two chambers on the left-hand side. On each side of the heart there is a pre-pumping chamber, the **atrium,** and a main pumping chamber, the **ventricle.** There is a right-sided and a left-sided ventricle. The muscle of the heart is called the **myocardium** (*myo* meaning muscle and *cardium,* being of the heart).

Blood drains from the body through the veins, collecting into two major veins called the **superior vena cava** (SVC) and the **inferior vena cava** (IVC) which drain into the right side of the heart. This blood arrives in the right atrium and is given a gentle pump through a one-way valve into the ventricle which then pumps the blood through another one-way valve into the lungs. Within the lungs, gas exchange occurs: oxygen is absorbed from the air we breathe in and carbon dioxide is released through the breath we exhale.

The blood then flows from the lungs to the left atrium. The left atrium gives a gentle pump and the blood passes through the mitral valve, a one-way valve, into the left ventricle which then contracts, squeezing blood through the aortic valve into the main artery of the body, the **aorta,** as it begins its journey around the body. The contraction of the left ventricle makes the blood flow through the arteries that we can feel pulsating under the skin.

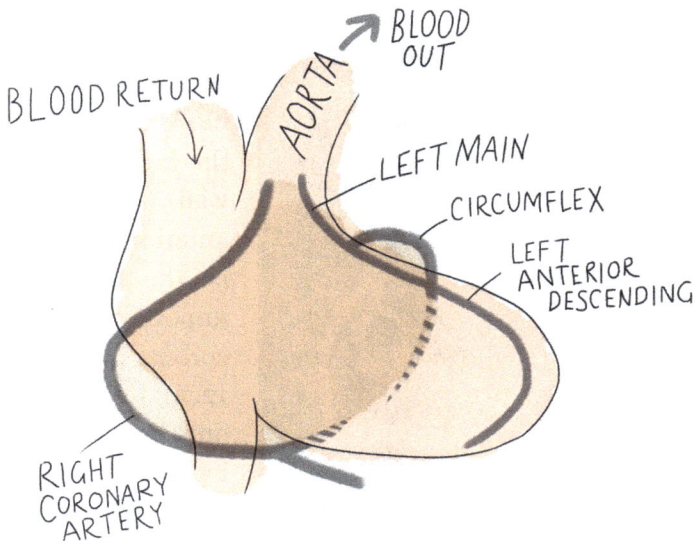

A schematic showing how the blood vessels wrap around the heart.

The coronary arteries arise from the aorta as it comes from the left ventricle. They are the first branches in the circulation.

It is useful to think of the arteries as the fuel lines supplying the cylinders of the car, transporting blood to different territories (pistons) of the heart muscle. This system consists of the **right coronary artery** and **left main coronary artery.** Within one centimetre, the left coronary artery divides into two main arteries: the **left anterior descending artery** which provides blood to the anterior surface of the heart, that is the surface nearest the chest wall, and the **circumflex artery** which supplies blood to the back of the heart or the surface of the heart nearest the spine. The **right coronary**

artery supplies the inferior surface of the heart or the surface that is nearest the diaphragm.

The terms 'right dominant' or 'left dominant' can be used in reference to the origin of the artery that supplies blood to the bulk of the inferior surface of the heart. This is generally from the right coronary artery but sometimes the right coronary is smaller and the circumflex is 'dominant', or bigger, supplying the majority of the inferior surface of the heart. This is called 'left dominant'. This becomes important in terms of the amount of the heart that may be affected by a blockage of the artery, the dominant artery providing blood to a larger territory.

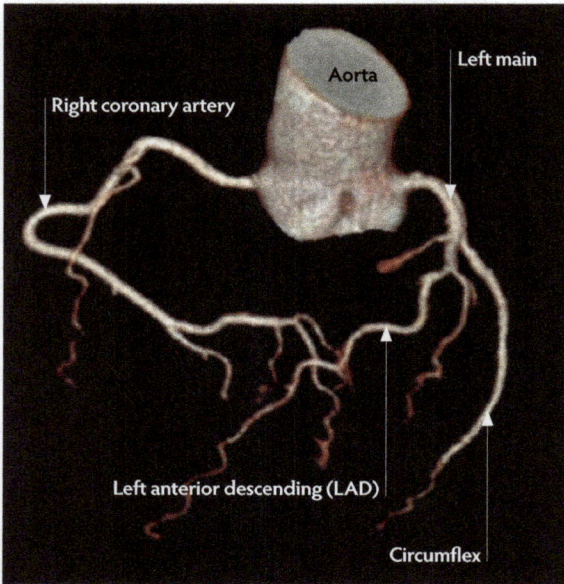

The coronary tree as seen on cardiac CT imaging.

The left anterior descending artery supplies blood to the anterior wall of the heart (nearest the chest wall). Most often, the left anterior descending artery is the largest and most important of the three main coronary arteries. It can be 12cm to 14cm long, while only two to five millimetres in diameter. This is little thicker than a pen refill, yet its blockage can be disastrous. A dominant right coronary artery can be approximately the same size and a non-dominant circumflex can be six to eight centimetres long and 1.5 to three millimetres in diameter.

The major arteries comprise fewer than 35cm in total length and fewer than five millimetres in diameter at their largest. A single build-up of plaque leading to a blockage may only be one centimetre in length. **This is not a system with a lot of redundancy, making it very vulnerable.**

Groundwork: the blood

It is important to be aware of the contents of the blood.

The heart pumps three to four litres of blood every minute.

The blood contains **red cells** which are carriers of **haemoglobin,** the oxygen-carrying substance which transports oxygen to the body's tissues. It is critical for the metabolism of the heart, or the normal working of the heart muscle, to receive a good supply of oxygen.

The other important components of the blood are the **platelets.** These small particles are central in forming clots or *thrombi* when damage is detected within the vascular system. Platelets stop the bleeding, for example, when we cut ourselves.

The blood also carries **nutrients** and fats such as **cholesterol.**

Coronary artery disease

Historically, it has not been possible to medically evaluate the coronary arteries in a well person. So, the first time that a problem with the arteries can be suspected is when symptoms (angina, shortness of breath or an acute coronary syndrome) present.

Angina is the term given to discomfort in the chest when pain is experienced in association with exertion. The term has its root meaning in a sense of strangulation.

Shortness of breath on exertion can indicate a lack of blood flowing to the heart. Under these circumstances the heart cannot work properly, pressures within the pumping chamber begin to rise with back pressure to the lungs and, consequently, the person experiences shortness of breath.

An **acute coronary syndrome** is the sudden development of a complete, or near complete, occlusion, or blockage, of a coronary artery. A lessened blood flow to a region of heart muscle results in damage. A complete blockage causes the death of that area of the heart muscle. This is called a **myocardial infarction** (*myo,* muscle, *cardiam,* heart; *infarction,* death by lack of blood flow). A near complete blockage, or 'unstable angina', puts strain on the heart and can be a forerunner to a complete blockage, or heart attack.

The medical term for 'heart attack', a full blockage or near-complete blockage of a coronary artery and its consequences, is **Major Adverse Coronary Event** or **MACE.** *(Heart attack is used in this book in the context of a major adverse coronary event and the terms will be used interchangeably.)*

Another important term in this discussion is **plaque.** This is the build-up of cholesterol, scavenger cells, scar tissue and calcium in the wall of the artery. The medical terminology for the build-up of these materials is **atherosclerotic plaque.** For simplicity, we will call this 'plaque' and at times simplify the process to a 'build-up of cholesterol in the arteries'. Plaque is localised. It occurs where wear and tear of the artery have led it to develop. *(Due to the importance of plaque in our discussions, a more detailed description of how plaque forms can be found at the end of this chapter.)*

The term ***coronary artery disease*** **describes the process of atherosclerosis or plaque build-up in the arteries that leads to impaired blood flow which causes symptoms or loss of function.**

CORONARY HEART DISEASE or heart disease affects around 1.4 million Australians and is the single leading cause of death in this country.

It kills 54 Australians each day, or one Australian every 27 minutes.

We know from observation that coronary artery disease is a patchy process. Autopsies on patients who have died from coronary artery disease have shown that generally a focal, localised area or lesion, or plaque has led to the life-ending event. Within the same artery, there can be areas that may not be diseased to the same extent, or even at all.

This is particularly significant when we consider sudden cardiac death. Most people can deal conceptually with the idea of some shortness of breath or chest pain on exertion. My own grandfather, for example, for a number of years had angina when he walked too far up the street or rushed while undertaking his daily activities. The real issue that concerns most of us is sudden cardiac death.

Could I please emphasise to the reader that these symptoms need to be taken seriously.

PLEASE, PLEASE, PLEASE seek immediate medical attention should you be affected by chest pain or unexplained shortness of breath.

Autopsies after sudden cardiac death from coronary artery disease show that about 60 percent of the culprit lesions or plaques have been **flow-limiting,** or tight, prior to the event that led to death and, hence, likely to have given a clue by way of a symptom such as chest pain or shortness of breath.

This leaves about 40 percent that has been **non-flow-limiting** before the event. In this situation, the person has no warning at all and so no chance to seek help before the event. This is the group in which death strikes suddenly and without warning, often in a seemingly fit and healthy person. **This is critical to our understanding of how we might be able to prevent death from coronary artery disease.**

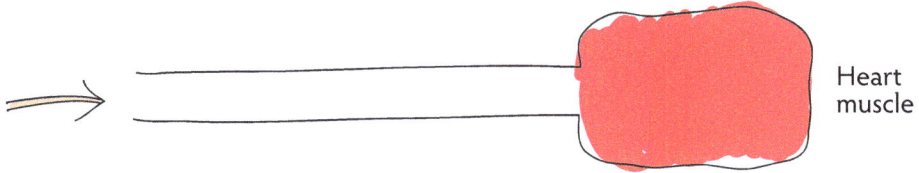

A schematic of a blood vessel supplying heart muscle.

Heart muscle

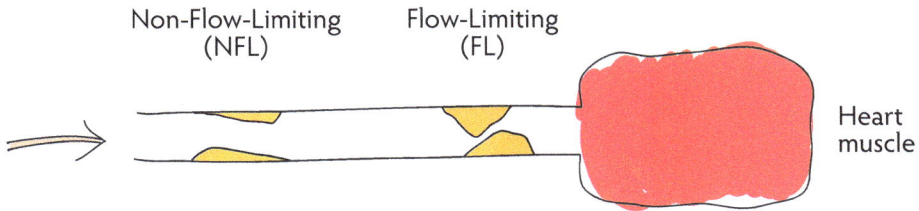

Non-Flow-Limiting (NFL)   Flow-Limiting (FL)

Heart muscle

A schematic showing build up of non-flow-limiting and flow-limiting plaque in the artery.

If we were to cut through the plaque (either the flow-limiting or non-flow-limiting) we would see similar components:

- the wall of the artery;

- the lumen (or inside space) of the artery;

- the cholesterol plaque which has built up and is beginning to intrude into the artery, and

- a fibrous cap that separates the plaque from the blood.

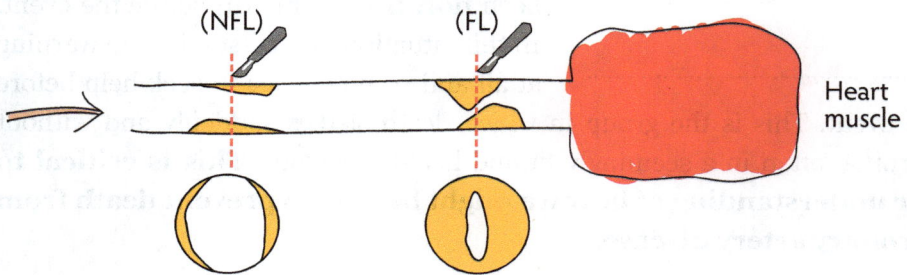

A schematic showing the components of non-flow-limiting and flow-limiting plaque are the same, just to a different extent.

The blood contains many different components. Importantly, there are platelets, those small particles responsible for the formation of a clot when any abnormality is detected in the inside lining of the artery. In an **unstable plaque,** rupture of the fibrous cap covering the build-up of cholesterol can occur. The blood comes into contact with the content of the plaque. The platelets, having rapidly detected the change, start to clump together to form a clot which may progress to a complete blockage of the artery.

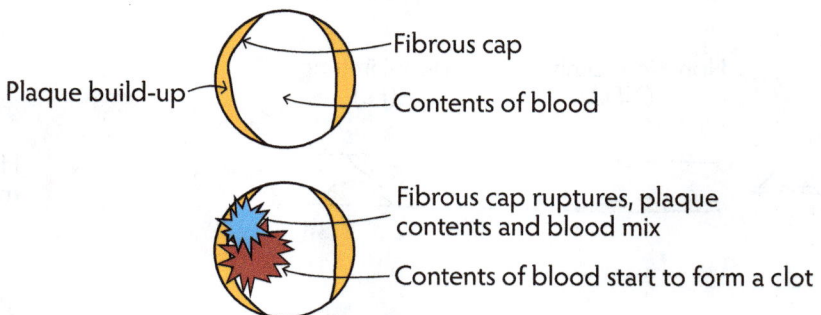

A schematic showing how, when the contents of the plaque come into contact with the contents of the blood, the body begins to form a clot.

This is so concerning because a non-flow-limiting plaque will give absolutely no symptoms, no clues, no warning. Even a microscopic tear in the fibrous cap of a plaque can lead to the formation of a clot, which can then rapidly block off that artery and be life-ending.

Ten to 15 percent of people who suffer a heart attack die[8,9], and many will have no prior warning.

AN INTERESTING POINT: If we were to suffer a cut, the platelets would clump at the site of the wound and save us from bleeding to death. In the setting of a ruptured plaque, the very thing platelets are meant to do can cause death.

IMPORTANT POINTS

- Detection and treatment of coronary artery disease, historically, has been related to the presence of symptoms or the occurrence of a major coronary event.

- Plaque is related to the build-up of cholesterol and other matter within the arteries. This build-up can be patchy, tending to occur where there are points of stress, weakness and/or vulnerability in the artery.

- Plaque can be flow-limiting (which generally, though not always, produces symptoms) or non-flow-limiting (which will cause no symptoms). However, in either case, unstable plaque can rupture and a clot, which can block the artery, can form very quickly. When a seemly fit and healthy person drops dead, during exercise, for example, it is often the case that the person had an unstable non-flow-limiting plaque rupture (and therefore, no symptoms before the life-ending event).

[1]   Abed MA, Khalil AA, Moser DK. Awareness of modifiable acute myocardial infarction risk factors has little impact on risk perception for heart attack among vulnerable patients. Heart Lung 2015;44:183-8.

[2]   Hoevenaar-Blom MP, Spijkerman AM, Boshuizen HC, Boer JM, Kromhout D, Verschuren WM. Effect of using repeated measurements of a Mediterranean style diet on the strength of the association with cardiovascular disease during 12 years: the Doetinchem Cohort Study. Eur J Nutr 2014;53:1209-15.

[3]   Lanas F, Avezum A, Bautista LE, et al. Risk factors for acute myocardial infarction in Latin America: the INTERHEART Latin American study. Circulation 2007;115:1067-74.

[4]   Celermajer DS, Chow CK, Marijon E, Anstey NM, Woo KS. Cardiovascular disease in the developing world: prevalences, patterns, and the potential of early disease detection. J Am Coll Cardiol 2012;60:1207-16.

[5]   Scandinavian Simvastatin Survival Study G. Randomised trial of cholesterol lowering in 4444 patients with coronary heart disease: the Scandinavian Simvastatin Survival Study (4S). The Lancet 1994;344:1383-89.

[6]   Ford I, Murray H, Packard CJ, Shepherd J, Macfarlane PW, Cobbe SM. Long-Term Follow-up of the West of Scotland Coronary Prevention Study. New England Journal of Medicine 2007;357:1477-86.

[7]   Sutton L, Karan A, Mahal A. Evidence for cost-effectiveness of lifestyle primary preventions for cardiovascular disease in the Asia-Pacific Region: a systematic review. Globalization and Health 2014;10:1-19.

[8]   Libby P, Ridker PM, Hansson GK. Progress and challenges in translating the biology of atherosclerosis. Nature 2011;473:317-25.

[9]   Aso S, Imamura H, Sekiguchi Y, et al. Incidence and mortality of acute myocardial infarction. A population-based study including patients with out-of-hospital cardiac arrest. Int Heart J 2011;52:197-202.

Now that we have a basic understanding of the heart, the next chapter looks at the current approach to discovering and treating coronary artery disease ... but before going there, we answer a couple of important questions about cholesterol and plaque.

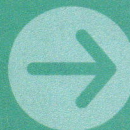

> what is cholesterol?

> how does plaque develop?

Throughout this book there are many references to plaque formation in the arteries and the build-up of cholesterol associated with plaque. It is important for you to have some understanding of what cholesterol is and the process of how plaque develops, as this will be useful in later discussions.

What is cholesterol?

Cholesterol is an organic (found in living systems) molecule. The word cholesterol has its origins in Greek: *chole* (bile) and *stereos* (solid) followed by the chemical suffix *-ol* for an alcohol.

Cholesterol is a waxy, fat-like substance. It makes up part of the cell membrane in all animals. It is also an important component of the material that wraps around nerve cells, acting a little like an electrical insulator. So, it is important and there is a lot of it around.

Cholesterol is also used to make a number of hormones: the hormones of the adrenal gland, which include the mineralocorticoids and the glucocorticoids. The mineralocorticoids help in the control of fluid balance and electrolytes in the body. The glucocorticoids are involved in the immune response. Cholesterol is also the basic building block for the sex hormones, progesterone, estrogen and testosterone, and their derivatives.

Cholesterol is also a precursor to the synthesis, or the making, of vitamin D.

All cells in the body are able to make cholesterol. However, we also consume foods that contain cholesterol. Of the ingested cholesterol, about 50 percent is absorbed into the body. There is variability in the cholesterol levels in the blood stream and this is generally genetically set such that even significant dietary efforts to alter cholesterol levels will rarely achieve greater than 15 percent changes in the measured blood cholesterol levels – a source of great frustration to many a patient!

Cholesterol is carried through the body by special proteins. There is a fair amount of complexity to this. However, in the simplest terms, there is a protein carrier that tends to take cholesterol from the liver and out to the tissues. This is called **low density lipoprotein** and is referred to as the 'bad' cholesterol. The protein that tends to carry cholesterol back to the liver is called **high density lipoprotein** and is denoted as the 'good' cholesterol.

The suggestion is that there is a **balance:** bad cholesterol puts cholesterol in the arteries and good cholesterol takes it away. Hence, the ratio of 'bad' cholesterol to 'good' cholesterol has historically been a mainstay of assessing the likelihood of a build-up of cholesterol in the arteries.

How does plaque develop?

PARTS OF THE ARTERY When we are born we have brand new healthy plaque-free arteries. The arteries are made up of three main layers: the inner layer, the middle layer and the outer layer.

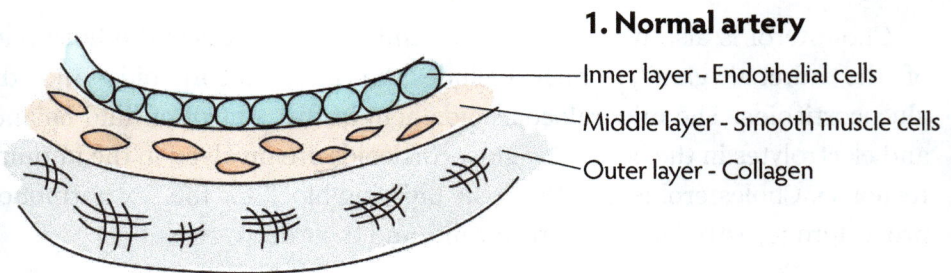

1. Normal artery

Inner layer - Endothelial cells

Middle layer - Smooth muscle cells

Outer layer - Collagen

The inner layer (*tunica intima* – meaning inner coat) is a smooth lining made from sheets of cells called the endothelium (*endo* – inside and *thelium* – skin). This amazing layer of cells makes sure the contents of the blood run smoothly through the blood vessel and do not stick or clump to the side wall of the artery. As well as acting as the 'Teflon lining' of the arteries, the endothelium also has a role in responding to stressors and strains within the artery and then communicates with the muscle layer of the artery to influence relaxation or contraction.

The middle layer (*tunica media* – middle coat) is predominantly made up of muscle cells. These are special muscle cells called **smooth** muscle. They are different to the muscles in your leg which are skeletal muscle (or, in your heart for that matter, which is cardiac muscle). Smooth muscles are not controlled by nerves in the way the skeletal muscles are but they respond to the automatic regulatory systems of the body. (You find smooth muscle in the wall of the stomach, gut, bladder and the ureters.) If you were to be frightened, the body's automatic (called the autonomic) nervous system would go into overdrive and pump adrenaline into the blood stream as well as activate the special nerves of the autonomic nervous system, leading to stimulation of the blood vessels' smooth muscle. As the smooth muscle contracts, it narrows the artery. As the same amount of blood is being pumped through narrower blood vessels, this results in an increase in blood pressure. *(This is over-simplified but it relates the basic idea.)* So this layer of the blood vessel has a significant influence on blood pressure regulation.

The outer layer (*tunica adventitia* – outside coat) is the main scaffold of the artery and is made up of collagen, the tissue that binds together almost all tissues in the body. The outer walls of the major arteries are, and have to be, very tough to deal with years of pulsating blood being forced through the body. Interestingly, the stretch and recoil of the walls of those big arteries act as a secondary pump for the body, maintaining flow between heart beats.

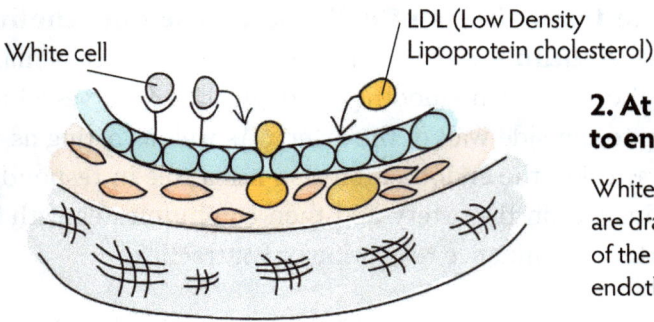

White cell

LDL (Low Density Lipoprotein cholesterol)

2. At site of damage to endothelium

White cells and cholesterol (LDL) are drawn into the artery at the site of the damage or trauma to the endothelium.

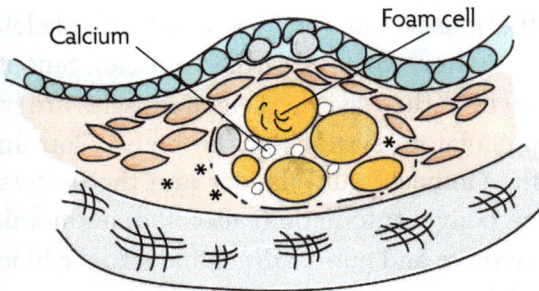

Calcium

Foam cell

3. Development of plaque

The white cells mature to macrophages that then consume the cholesterol, becoming 'foam' cells. These cells eventually burst, releasing enzymes that cause local scarring. Calcium moves into the scarred areas of plaque.

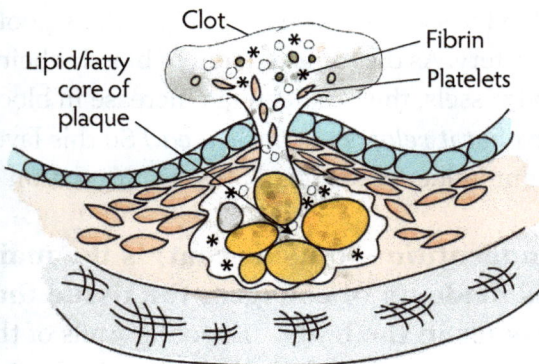

Clot

Lipid/fatty core of plaque

Fibrin

Platelets

4. Rupture of plaque and formation of clot (thrombosis)

A clot forms from the blood contents, reacting with the contents of the plaque when the plaque ruptures.

Now we know the parts of an artery, ***what happens that leads to the development of (coronary) atherosclerosis – or plaque?***

At a cellular level, minor damage to the endothelium, the lining of the artery, leads to 'activation' of the endothelium. This means the endothelium presents proteins to the bloodstream, which can attract and hold white cells (called leukocytes) which are the body's response to damage. The white cells are then drawn into the endothelium and from there, migrate into the space between the endothelial cells and the smooth muscle cells. At the same time, cholesterol is drawn into the wall of the artery, presumably as part of the healing process, as cholesterol is needed for the construction of cell membranes. The leukocytes then mature to cells that digest foreign material, the vacuum cleaners of the body. These mature cells are called macrophages [1,2].

The trouble is, the macrophages then start to clean up the low density cholesterol that has also come through the area of 'activated' endothelium.

The macrophages, or clean-up cells, gobble up the available cholesterol, becoming full and 'stuffed' with fat. They are then called foam cells. These foam cells age and eventually die, spilling their contents within the middle layer of the artery and extending toward the inner layer.

The spilt contents are the contents of the plaque, with free cholesterol and enzymes and cellular debris from the macrophages. The enzymes lead to microscarring and with cellular debris contribute to a matrix, or scaffold, that can subsequently become calcified.

This collection of cholesterol, scar tissue and calcium forms within the wall of the artery. **This is the plaque.** Ironically, it starts as a process to heal the artery. Yet, in some cases, it can progress to causing a problem, even death.

[1]   Libby P, Ridker PM, Maseri, A. Inflammation and Atherosclerosis. Circulation 2002;105;1135-43.

[2]   Bentzon JF, Otsuka F, Virmani R, Falk E. Mechanisms of Plaque Formation and Rupture. Circulation Research 2014;12:1852-66

HOPE FOR THE BEST OR EXPECT THE WORST...

We don't routinely treat 'low-risk' individuals, although up to 10 percent of that population may have an event. This is **hope for the best** as some of those individuals **will** have a MACE. Let's hope it is not someone we have reassured!

Conversely, we treat all of the individuals with 'high-risk', although up to 80 percent of them may have no problem at all in the next 10 years. This is **expecting the worst.**

Chapter 2 -
A current approach

> primary and secondary prevention

> population risk vs individual risk

> risk, association and causation

> understanding screening

Our approach to coronary artery disease tends mainly to focus on secondary prevention or dealing with the consequences of the disease: the symptoms and signs associated with a shortage of blood flowing to the heart, including shortness of breath, chest pain on exertion or an acute coronary syndrome.

On having diagnosed a patient, treatment is based on:

* understanding exactly where the problems are within the coronary arteries so that decisions can be made about whether re-establishing or improving blood flow with the use of technology such as stents or coronary artery bypass grafting is appropriate – **revascularisation,** and

* trying to prevent another event or a further problem occurring – **secondary prevention.**

Strategies to reduce the risk of a recurrence, include:

» the **use of medication**[1] to keep the platelets from clumping together and forming blockages in the arteries; aspirin is most commonly used for this;

» **reducing cholesterol levels**[1] to known targets associated with a significant improvement in outcome, often using cholesterol-lowering agents such as statins, and

» **life-style modifications**[2] that may reduce the risk, including exercise, weight loss, treatment of high blood pressure and/or diabetes, stopping smoking.

There is no question that secondary prevention is beneficial in reducing the recurrence of an event[3]. These patients clearly have a significant build-up of cholesterol in their arteries. The data around secondary prevention is very clear and I do not believe there is any need for alternative interpretations or strategies.

While my patients would tell you I adopt an almost boot camp mentality in my use of secondary prevention measures, from my perspective, the timing of secondary prevention is late in the process. You wouldn't want to die on your way to secondary prevention!

The problem is that the situation is not so sharply defined when it involves patients who have not yet had a problem. They may be at high-risk because of indicators such as cholesterol levels or blood pressure, or diabetes, or even smoking, yet they do not display any symptoms, nor have they been defined as having a problem. Even so, these patients may carry an increased risk. The treatment for that risk, **prior** to an event, is **primary prevention.**

My objective is to explore ways to avoid the first event. I believe that current primary prevention practice has scope for a *re-evaluation of our approach to risk assessment in individuals* before they even have a problem. For me, to prevent the chest pain or the heart attack in the first place is the Holy Grail of preventative cardiology.

The difficulty with primary prevention is that it involves the unrevealed:

- consideration of treatment before there is a clear indication as to whether or not an individual has a significant build-up of plaque within the arteries;
- whether or not the person has genuine high-risk features, and
- the probability of an event.

Defining risk

Within cardiology terminology, we define the risk of a coronary artery event as "low", "intermediate" or "high". A **low** risk is considered a less than 10 percent chance of a coronary event within 10 years. A **high** risk is considered a greater than 20 percent chance of an event within 10 years. An **intermediate** risk is between 10 and 20 percent risk of an event within 10 years.

This means that, if we were to take a group of 100 people who were high-risk and follow them for 10 years, 20 or more of those people would have a coronary event or symptom. If we introduced aspirin and a cholesterol-lowering tablet to reduce the risk of an event in this group of 100 then, statistically, we would be treating up to 80 people who were not going to have an event and perhaps did not need treatment. This has a significant impact on the way the effectiveness of that intervention is assessed. The statistical significance of assessing the effectiveness of primary prevention in this group is diluted by the people within the population who were not destined to have an event.

Similarly, if we were to take a group of 100 people with low risk of an event and follow them for 10 years, up to 10 of those individuals could have a coronary event and 90 would remain without any symptom or sign. Here again, the problem is: *How do we appropriately treat the 10 but not over-treat the 90?*

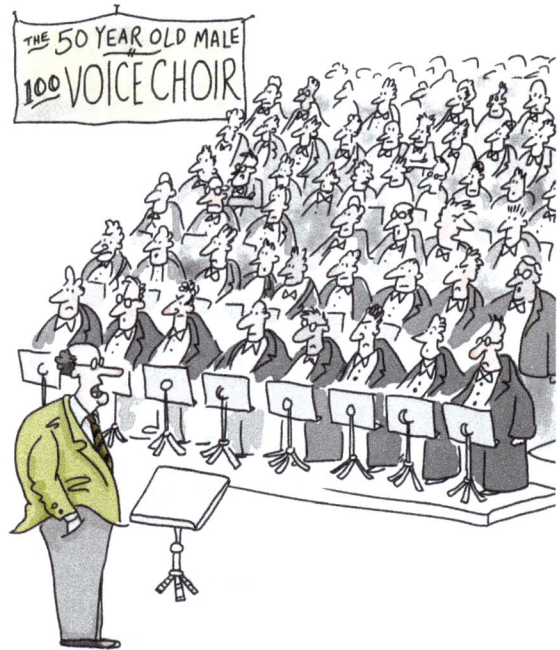

"OK guys, I've spoken to the doc and he says 10 to 15 of you will have a heart attack in the next 10 years. Could I just ask that it's not all the tenors?"

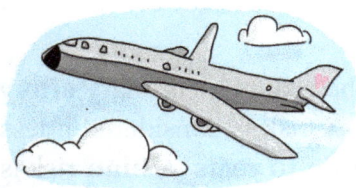

Interestingly, within the context of our medical classification, we are happy to refer to low risk as up to a 10 percent chance within 10 years and not consider treatment, even though this could be expressed as a one percent chance per annum of having a major event. How would you react if, the next time you booked a commercial airline flight, you were told there was a one percent per annum chance of being involved in a crash, or a 10 percent chance of being involved in a crash over your next 10 years of flying?

The way that we evaluate and calculate risk in individuals is based on **observational** data. This means that, over years, databases have been collated of features and factors found in individuals who have had coronary artery disease. The occurrence of those features and factors then lends weight to their being used as **predictors** for people **before they have an event.** This simply means that observational data collected on a large number of patients who have had heart attacks indicate that factors such as increasing age, being male, increased blood pressure, diabetic status and smoking all feature as **associations** to having had a coronary event.

This type of risk modelling, using multiple associations with observed outcomes, was first widely published and used by the **Framingham** Group[4]. This Framingham-type risk modelling continues to form the basis of our current risk assessment in primary prevention[5].

The interesting thing about this, of course, is that these factors are **associations,** and not necessarily **causations,** the mechanisms that actually cause the problem. This means that there can be people who are high-risk based on factors such as age, sex and cholesterol levels, yet never have an event. Conversely, there are people who would appear to score low on these risk calculators but still manage to have a coronary problem.

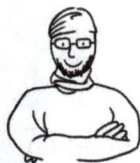

....

Understanding that our current risk evaluation is based on associations, and that those associations do not always necessarily have a direct link to the causation of the development of plaque within the arteries, is central to the discussion I wish to have throughout the remainder of this book.

....

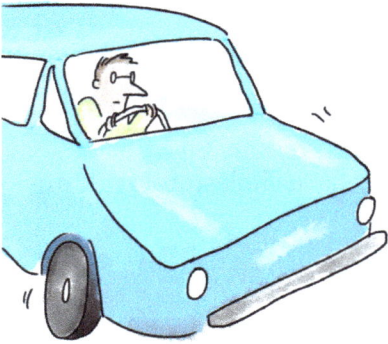

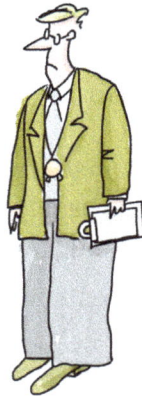

Let's look at this from outside the medical field. We know that speeding and alcohol consumption are significant associations of car accidents. However, we also know that people do drive over the speed limit with high alcohol levels, yet do not have an accident. Conversely, we know that people who drive safely can be involved in an accident.

This does not mean that driving within the speed limit and not consuming alcohol when driving are wastes of time. **It simply alters the risk profile.** It means that speed and alcohol are **associations** with having an accident. If they were **causations,** then every time someone sped or had consumed alcohol, that person would crash.

When it comes to the heart, being aware of your blood pressure and keeping it down, being aware of your cholesterol and dealing with it appropriately, undertaking regular exercise, not smoking and addressing other cardiovascular risks are all important for a safe journey through life. However, **on their own,** they offer **no guarantee** of avoiding a heart attack, although they are likely to **reduce** the **risk.** Remember the fun runner in the introduction: he was active, exercised regularly and had appropriate treatment for his blood pressure, yet that didn't protect him.

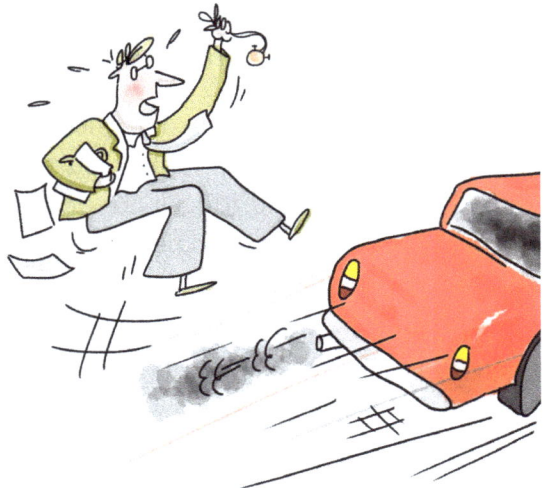

association vs causation

In discussing issues around **risk factor assessment** in relation to coronary artery disease, it is extremely important to be clear about the difference between **association** and **causation.**

Regularly, I need to advise patients that they have cholesterol build-up in their arteries.

Invariably I receive the reply,

- "But Doctor, my cholesterol is fine."
- "But Doctor, I exercise regularly."
- "But Doctor, I eat healthy food and keep my weight down."

These patients are expressing a belief which is **broadly accepted** but **universally misleading:** that certain factors, such as elevated cholesterol, lack of exercise, eating poorly or being overweight are the **direct causes** of coronary artery disease.

They are not the *causes;* they are *associations*.

If we were to return to our alcohol and driving example: alcohol is associated with an increased incidence of car accidents. Alcohol does not cause the car accident; it does not drive the car, yet alcohol can impair the driver's reflexes and assessment and **contribute** to that driver having an accident.

The actual **cause** of the accident may be approaching a sharp bend too quickly, a car in front stopping unexpectedly, changing the radio and losing concentration, or a dog running out on to the street.

In fact, a car accident is an excellent example when trying to understand association and causation. Multiple associations can be present such as alcohol, speeding, driver inexperience, poor weather. These associations, even when put together, do not necessarily mean that that car will be involved in an accident, just that there is **a higher risk.**

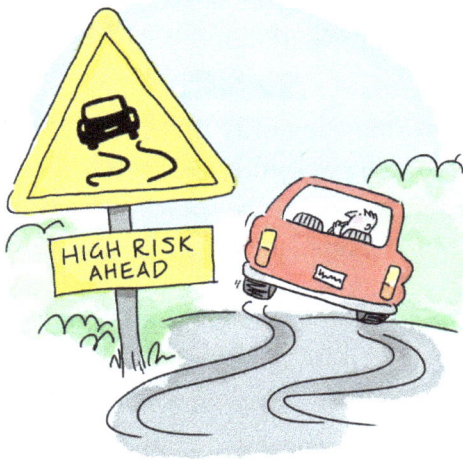

The reverse is true also. There may be no alcohol, no speeding, an experienced driver in good weather and yet, without any associations present, an accident occurs.

Our lack of understanding of the exact mechanisms of the development of coronary artery disease in a single individual, in a particular artery, at a particular location within the artery, means that our science around coronary artery disease is based on the science of **observation,** not the science of **mechanism.** Consequently, that science of observation leads to a clearer understanding of **association.**

The reason for highlighting this is that **there is a substantial gap between association and causation, and it is this gap that I hope to shed light on in subsequent chapters.**

We know, both from literature and from personal experience, of people with high cholesterol levels who do not have heart attacks, of people who exercise regularly and have a heart attack, seemingly out of the blue at a young age, of people who smoke, are overweight and do not exercise who live long lives without problems, and we see family clusters in which major adverse coronary events occur at a much higher frequency but not in all members.

Problems for primary prevention

Currently, the data that supports primary prevention is pretty thin[6-8].

Certainly in some **high**-risk groups, such as patients who have familial hypercholesterolaemia, there is no question that studies have shown primary prevention is beneficial. Hypercholesterolaemia is a genetic condition which gives rise to very elevated levels of cholesterol and is associated with a family history of premature coronary artery disease[9]. There is also reasonable data to support that high-risk patients, if appropriately selected, will benefit from intervention such as aspirin, lowered cholesterol, treatment of diabetes and lowered blood pressure, targeted in a primary prevention role[3,9].

The Achilles Heel of primary prevention arises in the **intermediate**-risk and **low**-risk populations. These groups, with the majority of the population being unlikely to have a problem, will need to be treated, accepting that they may not have an event over the next 10 or even 20 year period. Statistically, the effectiveness of a primary prevention regime, therefore, is markedly diluted and the cost of drugs, and side-effects associated with drugs, are spread across a large number of people who probably do not need them. The unfortunate consequence of this is that the 10 to 15 percent of people, who may appear to be at low to intermediate risk but will have an event and who may benefit, do not represent enough numbers to make these studies appear worthwhile or this intervention effective.

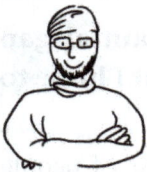

I will discuss in later chapters ways that we could become more precise around evaluating risk in the individual and therefore being more targeted in our approach to risk modification. This in turn, I believe, would make the process more efficient and more cost effective, and would improve the risk/benefit profile of the medications involved.

Screening using stress tests

Before moving on to that detail, however, I would like to mention a part of our current approach that I believe has some **significant limitations: stress testing as an indicator of coronary artery disease.** The exercise stress test, usually undertaken on a treadmill or a stationary exercise bike, is used to determine how blood is flowing through the arteries.

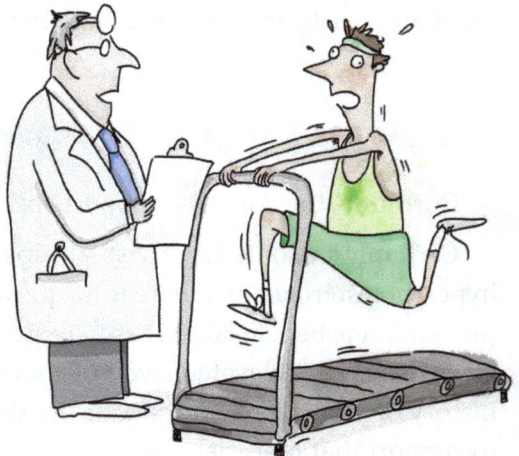

Health insurance companies and other agencies and organisations still use stress testing as an indicator of coronary artery disease. For example, there are guidelines within the Civil Aviation Safety Authority which dictate that pilots, beyond a certain age, should have regular stress testing. Until recently, this was a fair and reasonable thing to do, as it was, in fact, the only way we could try to unmask a problem within the arteries in a non-invasive and objective fashion. Available data suggest that if a patient performs well on a treadmill test without evidence of any problems, then his/her one year mortality, or risk of a major problem, is low[10]. Remember it was 'low' for the fun runner in the introduction.

By recalling our earlier discussion, you will appreciate that there is a limitation to this testing: that a significant amount of **cholesterol** or **atheroma** can build in the arteries **before** it actually leads to a narrowing and, therefore, before it shows any features on stress testing. Thus, it is fairly late in the process when it shows up. To a degree, that patient has run the gauntlet of a major event with potential rupture of the non-flow-limiting plaque which would remain undetectable because it causes no limitation to flow until the moment it ruptures.

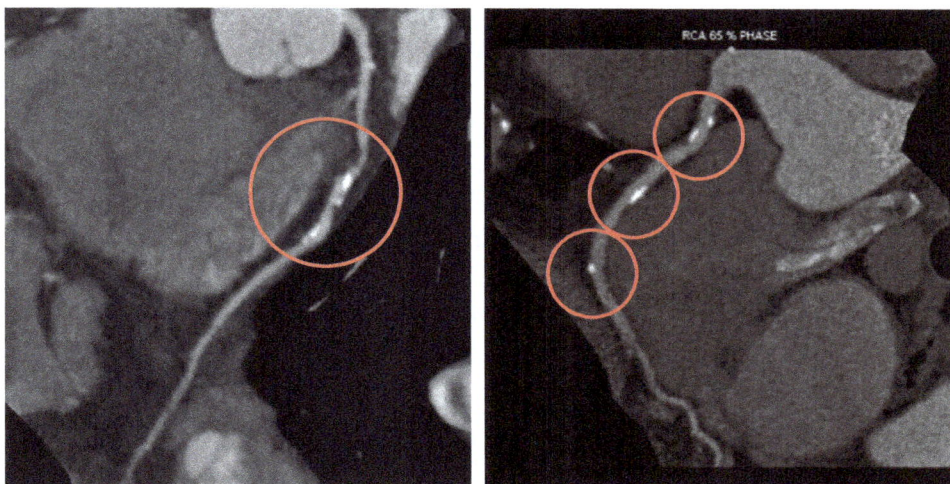

These are images from a cardiac CT scan done on a 61-year-old fireman who had had a "normal" exercise stress test, exercising for 12 minutes without problems. He still wanted more reassurance as he had a history of high blood pressure, and there was a family history of coronary disease and diabetes.

The scans clearly show a significant build-up of plaque that could not be picked up by the stress testing. This additional information allowed for appropriate risk management that otherwise would not have been undertaken.

I believe and hope some of the discussion that follows may reframe the approach to cardiovascular health assessment in situations for pilots, commercial drivers, emergency workers and the armed forces, and in insurance evaluations, as well as for the general population.

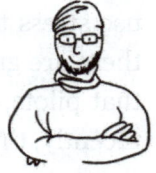

IMPORTANT POINTS

- Primary prevention aims at stopping someone from having a heart attack or developing heart problems. Scientific evidence to support this is not as strong as for secondary prevention, or preventing a second heart attack or recurrence of a problem.

- In evaluating for risk of an individual in primary prevention, we use associations which have been demonstrated in population studies. This presents an inherent problem as risk may be low for the population but is 100 percent for the individual who has an event.

- Individual screening using stress testing, as employed in some organisational settings, will pick up problems only late in the process of cholesterol build-up in the arteries.

[1]   Fleg JL, Forman DE, Berra K, et al. Secondary Prevention of Atherosclerotic Cardiovascular Disease in Older Adults: A Scientific Statement From the American Heart Association. Circulation 2013;128:2422-46.

[2]   Eckel RH, Jakicic JM, Ard JD, et al. 2013 AHA/ACC Guideline on Lifestyle Management to Reduce Cardiovascular Risk: A Report of the American College of Cardiology/American Heart Association Task Force on Practice Guidelines. Circulation 2014;129:S76-S99.

[3]   Abed MA, Khalil AA, Moser DK. Awareness of modifiable acute myocardial infarction risk factors has little impact on risk perception for heart attack among vulnerable patients. Heart Lung 2015;44:183-8.

[4]   Kannel WB, McGee D, Gordon T. A general cardiovascular risk profile: The Framingham study. The American Journal of Cardiology 1976;38:46-51.

[5]   Greenland P, LaBree L, Azen SP, Doherty TM, Detrano RC. Coronary artery calcium score combined with Framingham score for risk prediction in asymptomatic individuals. Jama 2004;291:210-5.

[6]   Sutton L, Karan A, Mahal A. Evidence for cost-effectiveness of lifestyle primary preventions for cardiovascular disease in the Asia-Pacific Region: a systematic review. Globalization and Health 2014;10:1-19.

[7]   Scandinavian Simvastatin Survival Study G. Randomised trial of cholesterol lowering in 4444 patients with coronary heart disease: the Scandinavian Simvastatin Survival Study (4S). The Lancet 1994;344:1383-89.

[8]   Ford I, Murray H, Packard CJ, Shepherd J, Macfarlane PW, Cobbe SM. Long-Term Follow-up of the West of Scotland Coronary Prevention Study. New England Journal of Medicine 2007;357:1477-86.

[9]   Watts GF, Sullivan DR, Poplawski N, et al. Familial hypercholesterolaemia: a model of care for Australasia. Atheroscler Suppl 2011;12:221-63.

[10] Shaw LJ, Peterson ED, Shaw LK, et al. Use of a prognostic treadmill score in identifying diagnostic coronary disease subgroups. Circulation 1998;98:1622-30.

The next chapter presents several case studies to help further set the scene.

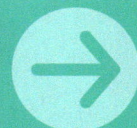

Chapter 3 -
A picture paints a thousand words

> several very different case studies

One of the key tools to my approach to primary prevention is to use the latest technology available to scan the heart. We will go into detail in later chapters but for the moment it is enough to appreciate that, by scanning the heart, I can obtain as much information as possible about the condition of the arteries of the patient's heart by looking at the arteries literally to see what is going on.

As 'a picture paints a thousand words', here are some 'patient pictures' as examples.

KAREN was a 60-year-old woman who came to see me for cardiovascular risk stratification. She was generally fit and well, not on any regular medication and there was no history of premature coronary artery disease in her family. Her cholesterol profile was:

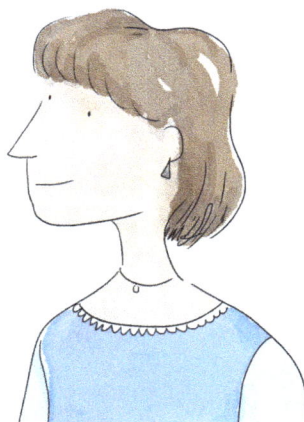

Total Cholesterol (TC)	9.1	ideally < (less than) 5.0 mmol/l
Triglycerides (TG)	2.0	ideally <2.0 mmol/l
High Density Lipoprotein (HDL)	2.1	ideally > (greater than) 1.0 mmol/l
TC to HDL ratio	4.3	ideally <4.0 ratio
Non HDL	7.0	ideally <4.0 mmol/l
Low Density Lipoprotein (LDL)	6.1	ideally <2.5 mmol/l

This was her Australian cardiovascular disease risk factor calculator result.

This was not a good result. The calculator estimated her risk at greater than a 15 percent chance of an event in the next five years, or over 30 percent in 10 years. This was a very high risk, so high that she had a red thermometer!

It transpired that, over the years, each time Karen had visited her doctor, she had been given a script for a cholesterol-lowering tablet; each time she had suffered side-effects and had stopped taking the tablets within weeks. We spoke at length about using CT to image the heart, to provide more detail regarding the 'health' of her arteries. Karen agreed as she was eager to see what was really going on.

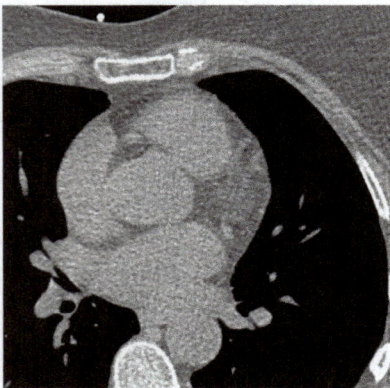

This is the scan result for Karen. Her coronary calcium score was zero. There was no evidence of plaque build-up at all, despite her cholesterol levels. We did not undertake further evaluation.

This result was a fantastic relief to Karen who had been stressed by the desire of her local doctor to have her on a cholesterol-lowering tablet, not withstanding the side-effects she suffered. She was caught between the fear of an event and the side-effects of medication.

Based on the above scan, I could reassure her that all the available research suggests that the presence of a zero calcium score was a very low-risk feature, likely to represent a risk of event of less than one percent in 10 years (all things being equal). We discussed this at some length and agreed on a plan of management. As there was no evidence of plaque, there appeared to be no benefit for her in taking a statin or aspirin. However, we acknowledged that the literature's suggestion of a very low risk of an event over 10 years might not be the situation in her case because of the higher than average cholesterol level. So to err on the side of caution, we decided to repeat the scan in five years and reconsider treatment based on that next result.

A demonstrated low risk of event informed the immediate medication decision, which was backed up by a plan for ongoing surveillance. Karen was happy with the outcome.

....

TWO SISTERS, TRACEY and BECK, came to see me. Both had elevated cholesterol levels and there was a family history of premature coronary artery disease. They were in their early 50s and neither wanted to take cholesterol-lowering medication unless it were really necessary. Their cholesterol profiles were:

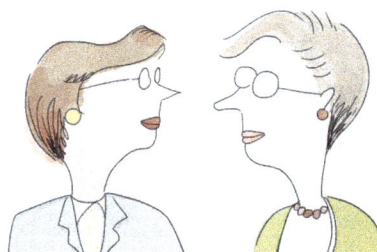

Tracey:

Total Cholesterol (TC)	8.2	ideally < (less than) 5.0 mmol/l
Triglycerides (TG)	2.2	ideally <2.0 mmol/l
High Density Lipoprotein (HDL)	1.0	ideally > (greater than) 1.0 mmol/l
TC to HDL ratio	8.2	ideally <4.0 ratio
Non HDL	7.2	ideally <4.0 mmol/l
Low Density Lipoprotein (LDL)	6.2	ideally <2.5 mmol/l

Beck:

Total Cholesterol (TC)	10.6	ideally < (less than) 5.0 mmol/l
Triglycerides (TG)	12.5	ideally <2.0 mmol/l
High Density Lipoprotein (HDL)	0.8	ideally > (greater than) 1.0 mmol/l
TC to HDL ratio	13.3	ideally <4.0 ratio
Non HDL	9.8	ideally <4.0 mmol/l

(LDL) unable to be measured accurately because of high TG

For both sisters, the Australian cardiovascular disease risk calculator suggested a risk of an event of greater than 15 percent in five years. After discussing the pros and cons of using cardiac CT, both sisters proceeded with the testing.

These are the results:

Tracey

This is a zero calcium score and suggests a low risk of coronary event in the next 5 to 10 years.

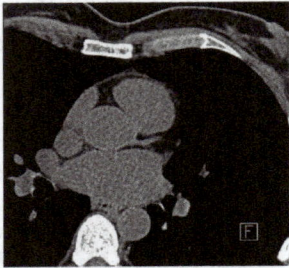

Tracey's scan for coronary calcium score

Beck

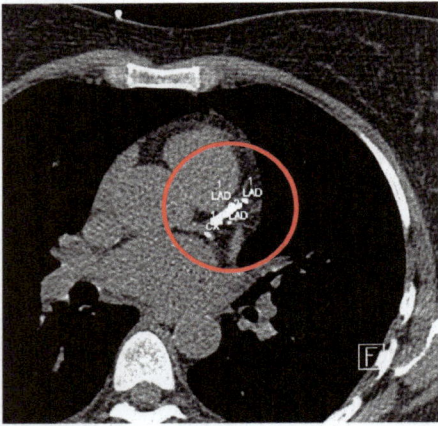

Beck's coronary calcuim

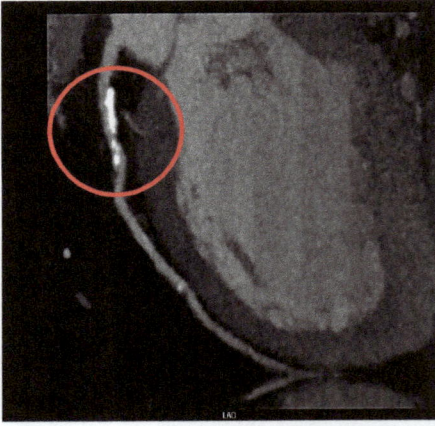

Left anterior descending artery

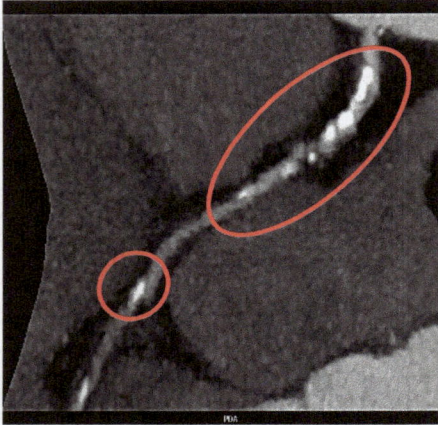

Right coronary artery

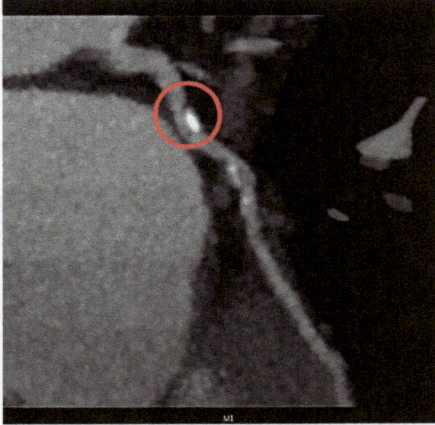

Circumflex artery

56

For Beck, the calcium score was over 1000. This was very high and, in comparison with 100 women of the same age taken randomly from the population, would be at least in the highest five (above the 95th percentile), perhaps even the highest.

Even without experience at looking at cardiac CT images, it can be seen that the pictures clearly show a significant build-up of plaque in all three arteries.

Beck's scans suggest very **high-risk** features.

These may be two sisters with the same family history and both with elevated cholesterol. However, the health of their arteries couldn't be more different. And no, I can't explain it.

Nonetheless, the information was clear and allowed a management strategy based on **exactly** what was seen to be going on in the arteries, not a best guess based on a population-based **probability** of what may be going on. *(The importance of this will become much clearer in subsequent chapters.)*

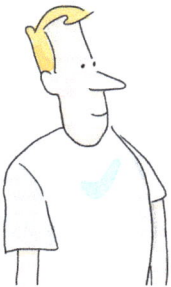

....

TONY was 63 years old when he came to see me. He was proactive about his health and wanted to be as clear as possible about his cardiac risk. When I saw him, he was taking a cholesterol-lowering tablet although it was a low dose and not aimed at the targets for a high-risk patient. He was not on aspirin. Interestingly, at his own initiation, he had undergone two treadmill stress tests (through another centre) in the previous two years and had been reassured everything was fine. When he came to see me he just wanted as much information as possible to be clear he was addressing his cardiovascular risk appropriately. This was his lipid profile:

Total Cholesterol (TC)	3.6	ideally < (less than) 5.0 mmol/l
Triglycerides (TG)	1.4	ideally <2.0 mmol/l
High Density Lipoprotein (HDL)	0.7	ideally > (greater than) 1.0 mmol/l
TC to HDL ratio	5.1	ideally <4.0 ratio
Non HDL	2.9	ideally <4.0 mmol/l
Low Density Lipoprotein (LDL)	2.2	ideally <2.5 mmol/l

These numbers look pretty good, so why worry? Well, we spoke at length and Tony was eager to proceed to imaging of his heart arteries for his own peace of mind.

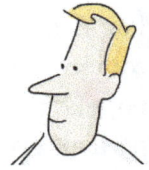

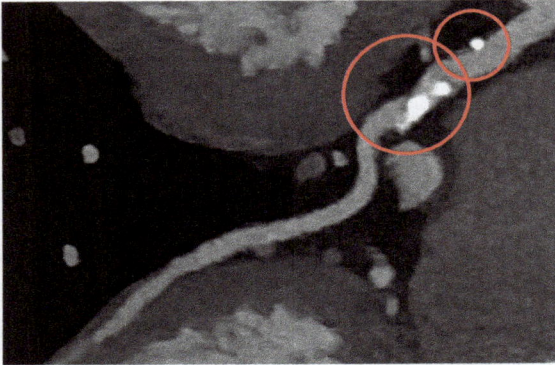

Tony's right coronary artery

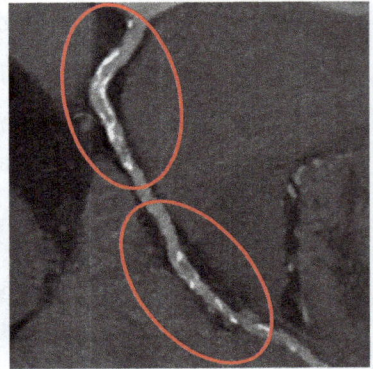

His circumflex artery

As you can see he has significant build-up. In fact, his calcium score was so high, it fell above the 90th percentile for his age group. The features were of very high risk for a coronary event.

With this information, we have, of course, commenced aspirin; we have increased his lipid-lowering therapy and improved his lipid profile in keeping with current guidelines. It has also been valuable in providing a focus to maximise lifestyle changes. The other important factor is that Tony is now well educated. Should there be **any** symptom that could be related to his heart, he knows to present for medical attention immediately. This education on its own could be life saving.

Tony was very pleased to have gone through the testing and to be better informed. There is no question that we have been able to improve his therapy in relation to his actual risk based on the state of his arteries. He realised that the stress tests had told him that he was 'fit' but had not told him the 'fitness' of his arteries.

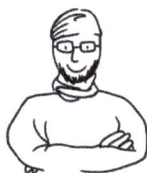

I found it interesting that Tony had been given a statin for cardiovascular risk but had not been given aspirin. Debate surrounds the role of the broad use of aspirin for reducing risk in primary prevention[1]. The current recommendation is that it is not indicated. This is also the case in diabetes[2]. Tony's situation seemed odd; either he had an increased risk of heart attack or stroke and deserved treatment, or not. To use one but not the other seems to me like not using the seat belt because your car has an airbag. Why wouldn't you use all the safety features?

Data suggest that aspirin is beneficial for a patient who is having a heart attack or who has had a heart attack[3,4]. So why wouldn't you give it to patients who seem to be at high risk of an event?

The answer is because there is no evidence it is beneficial if given to patients before an event. It seems logical to me that if you could give aspirin to the patient who is about to have a heart attack, it should help that person in the same way as a patient who has had a heart attack.

Later, I will discuss how we can better identify those high-risk patients by scanning their hearts, a technique not used in the studies looking at the role of aspirin in primary prevention. I will also talk about how the evidence base that we use in medicine to help decision-making and to formulate guidelines may have limitations. I hope to give enough information for YOU to decide if YOU would take aspirin if YOU were at high risk of a heart attack. I know I would!

STEVE was in his late 60s when he came to see me. He was slim, kept active and was generally well. This was his lipid profile:

Total Cholesterol (TC)	5.6	ideally < (less than) 5.0 mmol/l
Triglycerides (TG)	0.4	ideally <2.0 mmol/l
High Density Lipoprotein (HDL)	2.5	ideally > (greater than) 1.0 mmol/l
TC to HDL ratio	2.2	ideally <4.0 ratio
Non HDL	3.1	ideally <4.0 mmol/l
Low Density Lipoprotein (LDL)	2.9	ideally <2.5 mmol/l

This looks fairly unremarkable. When I plugged his features into the Australian cardiovascular disease calculator, he had a risk of six percent of an event in five years. This is considered a low risk and was represented by a green bar.

He was concerned, however, because his brother, who was of similar build and without significant cardiac risk, had required by-pass grafting months earlier. Steve wanted to know if he were at risk. After we discussed using

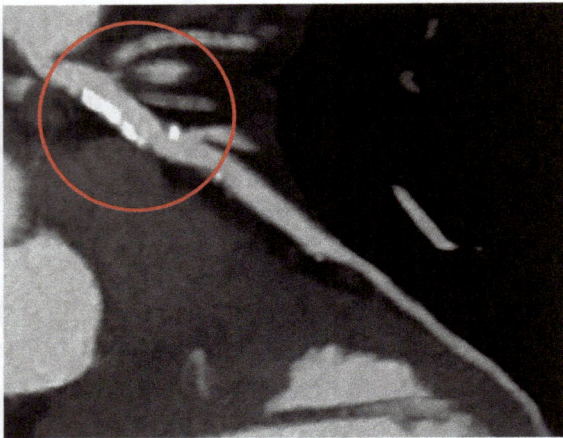

cardiac CT imaging to obtain more information, Steve wished to proceed with the testing.

This image clearly demonstrates calcific (bright white) and non-calcific (dark) plaque. His calcium score was over 250 and, as can be seen from the image, there is significant plaque in the proximal part of the artery. My evaluation of the findings was that, left unattended, the plaque features suggested a greater than 20 percent risk of a cardiac event in 5 to 10 years, considerably higher than his risk calculator.

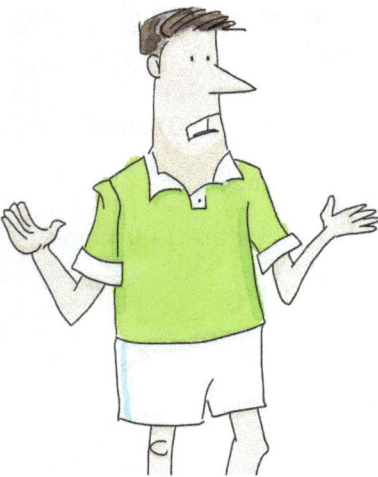

I spoke with Steve, reviewing his scan with him and explaining the findings. My feeling was that the risk features were high enough to warrant consideration of statin therapy and aspirin, to modify risk.

He was happy to go on medication for prevention, together with his current healthy lifestyle. However, in Australia, his lipid profile didn't allow the prescription of a statin to be supported by the Pharmaceutical Benefits Scheme. This meant that he had to self-fund the medication which, with the information he then had, he was more than happy to do.

PENNY was 52 years old when she came to see me. She was generally well and on no medication. She was a non-smoker and didn't have elevated blood pressure. She was concerned, however, because she had a terrible family history of premature coronary disease. Her lipid profile was:

Total Cholesterol (TC)	6.1	ideally < (less than) 5.0 mmol/l
Triglycerides (TG)	0.6	ideally <2.0 mmol/l
High Density Lipoprotein (HDL)	2.1	ideally > (greater than) 1.0 mmol/l
TC to HDL ratio	2.1	ideally <4.0 ratio
Non HDL	4.0	ideally <4.0 mmol/l
Low Density Lipoprotein (LDL)	3.7	ideally <2.5 mmol/l

If we put these results into the Australian cardiovascular disease risk calculator, we see Penny's risk is estimated at one percent in five years and she gets a green indicator.

The important thing to remember here is that a risk calculator doesn't predict the risk for an **individual** patient. Rather, it provides the rate events occur in a **group** of 100 individuals with the same characteristics. This does not tell us who of the 100 will have the event.

Penny was well informed when she came to see me. She had already had a significant discussion with her general practitioner and had looked at my website to obtain information about scanning the heart. Her husband, who came with her, also decided to have his heart scanned. He was about the same age, with a similar lipid profile, had borderline blood pressure and had a bit of weight on his tummy. He was the one who looked as if he might have the unhealthy arteries.

This was Penny's calcium score image and results:

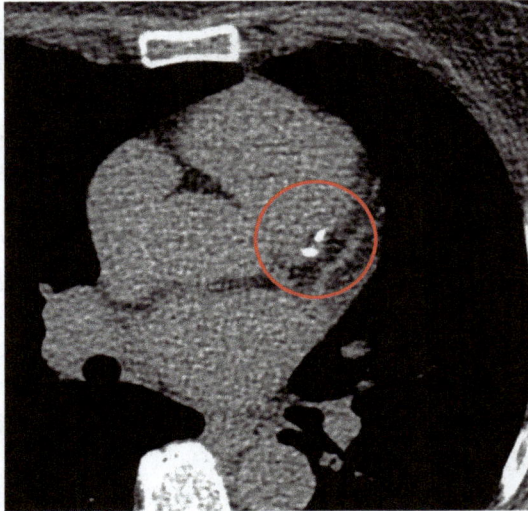

	Scoring Results : Agatston Score Protocol			
	LAD	LCX	RCA	Total Coronaries
Score	71.45	30.64	141.35	243.44
#ROI's	2	2	14	18
AreaSq (sq.mm.)	17.86	12.77	46.22	76.85

Her score of 243 is high for a young woman. For her age, the 90th percentile is 65! This result is three to four times higher, suggesting that Penny was probably the one out of 100, the one percent.

Although the results brought Penny to tears when she first heard this news, as the significance of having this knowledge sank in, she calmed down. There was no narrowing in the arteries and there had been no damage to the heart. And we had found what we had been looking for – to see if she had the same issues as others in her family. Although she did, **we had found the brake cylinder that was about to fail** *before* **the accident!**

We were able to institute therapy. For her, we were ahead of the game. There is little doubt that Penny found this process confronting but invaluable. And just to compete the story, her husband had a zero calcium score!

IMPORTANT POINTS

This series of patients includes examples of:

- high cholesterol and no evidence of problems in the arteries;
- high cholesterol and lots of plaque in the arteries;
- unremarkable lipid profile and high-risk features in the arteries, and
- family history with varying outcomes.

There is considerable complexity around these issues but I will discuss them in more detail throughout the book so that you will be equipped with the information you need to *Plan (not to have) Your Heart Attack*.

[1]   Cleland JG. Is aspirin useful in primary prevention? European heart journal 2013:eht287.

[2]   Nelson MR, Doust JA. Primary prevention of cardiovascular disease: new guidelines, technologies and therapies. Med J Aust 2013;198:606-10.

[3]   Berger JS, Brown DL, Becker RC. Low-dose aspirin in patients with stable cardiovascular disease: a meta-analysis. Am J Med 2008;121:43-9.

[4]   Collaborative meta-analysis of randomised trials of antiplatelet therapy for prevention of death, myocardial infarction, and stroke in high-risk patients. BMJ 2002;324:71-86.

The next chapter asks: "Is medical opportunity knocking on the door?" While there is no question that evidence-based medicine is the appropriate way to advance medical care, could rigid adherence to this approach hinder good medicine?

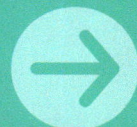

Chapter 4 -
The art of good medicine

> the discrepancy between evidence-based trials
and medical opportunity

Our discussion brings us to a point where there is an obvious medical opportunity to be ahead of the game in regard to an individual's coronary risk, by using a combination of the standard risk factor modelling and cardiac CT imaging. Why, then, is this not being done on a regular basis?

Cardiac CT imaging is not widely used in primary prevention because **no randomised double-blind control trials exist to demonstrate that it is beneficial in improving outcomes for the individuals who are scanned compared with a control group.** This is an absolutely critical point when it comes to understanding the slow uptake of a technology that would appear to be incredibly useful in the management of patients in a primary preventative role. The lack of clear-cut trial data means that there is a lack of an evidence base to support using cardiac CT imaging in primary prevention assessments.

Current medical practice, by and large, is founded on the concept of evidence-based medicine[1]. This means that patient management guidelines or recommendations which are put together by speciality groups or organisations are founded on a clear understanding that there has been appropriate research in an area and an unmistakable demonstration that the intervention being discussed has, without question, been shown to be beneficial.

There is absolutely **no question** that evidence-based medicine **is** the appropriate way to advance medical care. It is a solid foundation that demonstrates clearly that what we are doing has been proven to be safe and beneficial when applied to clinical practice[1]. All doctors need to be aware of the importance of evidence-based medicine in all undertakings in patient care. In no way should it be diminished.

Evidence-based limitations

While the importance of a body of evidence in any area of medicine helps to guide best practice and appropriate management for an individual, **sole reliance** on this approach presents potential limitations.

FIRSTLY, there is enormous complexity in medical/biological systems and sometimes multiple variables can be extremely difficult to assess in a large population over a long time.

For example, there is good evidence that aspirin is beneficial for patients who have had a myocardial infarction[2,3]. If, however, we were to ask, *Is it beneficial for patients who are left handed, wear spectacles and who are blond?* then, because those criteria were not necessarily tested during the trial, we would not have a definitive answer and, therefore, would not have a strong evidence base if we were dealing with a patient who was left handed, wore glasses and was blond. We would have to make an assumption and, as soon as we do that, by definition, we step away from evidence. This creates a rigidity to evidence-based medicine as it will never address all variables or questions in the evaluation of an individual with characteristics distinct from the average.

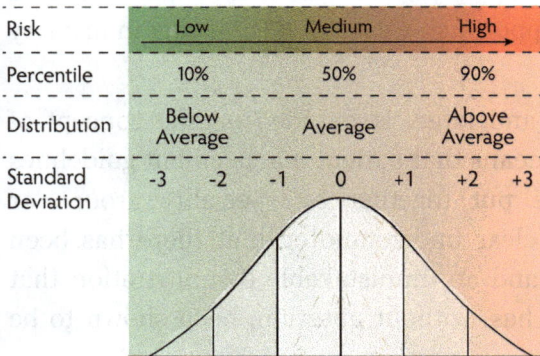

Risk	Low		Medium		High	
Percentile	10%		50%		90%	
Distribution	Below Average		Average		Above Average	
Standard Deviation	-3	-2	-1	0	+1	+2	+3

SECONDLY, the individual patient may be different to the evaluation of the averaged population from which the information has come. Populations will demonstrate a distribution curve which will have an average or mean but also have lower, as well as upper, extremes. The average results of the population may not be as applicable to the individuals at each end of the population spread. For example, we might undertake a study that gives us an average shoe size for adult males but is that applicable to our patient if he is a professional basketball player or a jockey?

THIRDLY, evidence-based medicine may have the limitation

that the study has not been done and may never be done. This was highlighted in a paper published in the *British Medical Journal* in 2003 (Smith GC, Pell JP. *Parachute use to prevent death and major trauma related to gravitational challenge: systematic review of randomised controlled trials*[4]). It has affectionately become known as the "Parachute Paper".

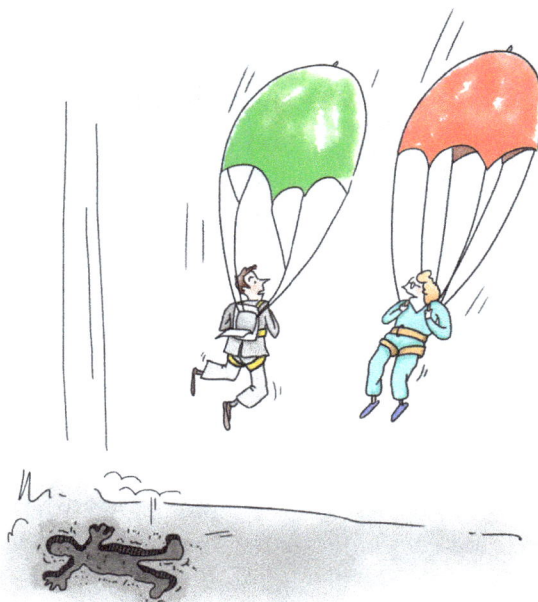

man: "Wow! What was that?"
woman: "Oh, that's Simon. First time jumper. Refused to use a parachute. Said there was no evidence that they worked!"

In this paper the authors set out very clearly, within the appropriate and correct constructs of evidence-based medicine, that, **because of a clear lack of data** (specifically, randomised control trials surrounding the use of parachutes), **one can conclude that parachutes do not work.** I believe the 'man on the street' quite happily accepts that parachutes do work. I think the 'man on the street' also accepts that it is not an absolute requirement for us to have a double-blind randomised control trial in which we would take a group of people with parachutes and push them out of a plane and then take, as the control group, another group of people without parachutes and push them out of a plane and compare the results!

This is a situation in which the randomised, double-blind controlled study has not been done. Common sense and, of course, an ethics committee, would never allow it to proceed. Clearly, it is a situation in which the observational data is reliable enough to draw a conclusion. However, it is an important reminder that **there will always be trials that have not been, and will not be, done and so there will be gaps in our evidence base within medicine.**

The first use of penicillin was so dramatic that its initial use was not randomised. The first 10 patients to receive an aortic valve (heart valve) replacement died before leaving hospital. This didn't stop the pursuit of a common sense solution to a clear problem. Further, there has never been a randomised controlled trial to assess the safety and efficacy of general anaesthesia. Think about it. Does general anaesthesia work? To find out, would you be prepared to be randomised in a study in which you could undergo surgery without anaesthesia? **The shortage of evidence-based studies did not stop these treatments from becoming commonly accepted.**

FOURTHLY, a study which has been undertaken to answer a question can, in retrospect, be seen to be **inadequately designed** and so does not fulfil all the requirements of its initial intention. This means that an evidence base can be constructed from research work which offers some, but not necessarily all, insight into a particular situation.

If I could illustrate this with an example. A study could be undertaken to look at the effect of reducing road accidents by reducing alcohol consumption. The study could be set up in controlled circumstances. There may be one group who drinks alcohol and a control group who does not drink. This sounds like a very simple way to demonstrate that alcohol consumption would make a difference to the likelihood of a crash. The test could be undertaken on a regulated track and one would think that the data would clearly demonstrate that the individuals consuming alcohol would have a greater rate of accident.

Yet, if:

- all cars were limited to a top speed of 40km/hr because the investigators didn't want the risk of high speed accidents, and

- alcohol consumption were limited to one standard drink because the investigators were teetotallers and considered this a significant amount,

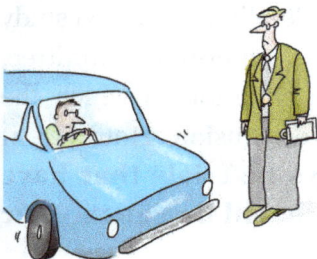

then it is possible that the effect of alcohol on driving error may be significantly diminished by the slow speed and the low blood alcohol levels, such that the group who had consumed alcohol may not have a statistically significant increase of events compared with the control group.

If

- no speed limit were imposed;

- the participants were instructed to complete the track circuit as quickly as possible, and

- they were instructed to drink to a blood alcohol level of greater than 0.05 percent (the legal limit in Australia),

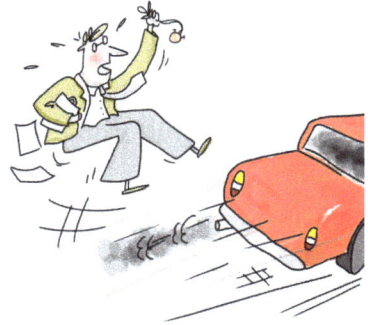

then there would be a clear difference due to the effect of alcohol.

In the above situation, the study design may actually lead to an outcome in which the full impact of an intervention (alcohol) is not appreciated statistically. The study may have been undertaken with meticulous attention to scientific rigour; it may have had unquestionable statistical analysis; it may tick all the required boxes to achieve merit for publication. This is very important because if this piece of information then forms part of the evidence base within that area of medicine, it brings with it the limitations of that trial design and results. In this situation, it would be possible to argue that under controlled conditions with good scientific rigour and extensive statistical analysis, alcohol was not shown to increase risk of accident. Only on looking deeper into the study would it become apparent that flaws with the study design (limiting speed and an inadequate alcohol consumption) might have lead to a misleading conclusion. Editorial comments during publication may flag these shortfalls but sometimes it is not until some time later that the limitation is recognised and the headline of the study remains to permeate more effectively than its detail.

This occurred with a major study designed specifically to demonstrate the value of cardiac CT imaging in risk assessment. The trial was called the St Francis Heart study[5]. The consequence of its failure has effectively applied a handbrake to the broader use of cardiac CT. I will discuss the study in more detail later *(refer to Chapter 16)*. Remember, also, that the best observational tool is the 'retro-spectroscope' and, in this situation, it is reasonable to expect that a study to explore a new area may not be designed as well as it could have been, because there was not enough knowledge at the time to guide the process.

FIFTHLY, time can erode 'evidence' in some situations as nothing stays the same. Think of the 'evidence' about mobile phones 20 years ago. Who would have said that most people would be carrying one now and more importantly, who would have imagined the functionality of smart phones today?

Time and changes in technology can move the goal posts in medicine, too. For example, when we advise patients that a new valve should last 15 years, what we are really saying is that valves that were made and implanted 20 plus years ago have been lasting around 15 years in the patients who received them. We can say that because it took a few years to become comfortable with the results, then time has been needed to track outcomes. What we don't really know is if the experience gained and the technology developed over the past 20 years mean that the valves currently being produced will last longer.

The same changing technology is impacting on CT imaging in regard to image quality. Radiation doses and even contrast doses are now out of date based on the leading-edge machines, which are improving with each tick of the clock and technological advance. This rapidly changing landscape of technology means it is very hard, almost impossible, to have robust 'current' data, as each time a study is started the new iteration of technology moves the goal posts again, and again, and again. This is good for the patient but not so good for having an evidence base that truly reflects an up-to-date situation.

PENULTIMATELY, studies can appear to provide conflicting information. Perhaps a recent trial proves the opposite results to a trial that we have relied on for some years. Which trial do we believe? Was the new one with better computing and technology more reliable or was the old trial more reliable?

This can be a difficult issue. In cardiology for example, niacin, or vitamin B3, has been used for many years to manage lipid levels in the blood. Some years ago, in a trial called the HATS[6] trial, niacin, together with a statin, showed significant outcome benefit. However, more recently, a trial called the AIM-HIGH[7] trial suggested niacin was not helpful and could be potentially harmful. The 'headline results' of the AIM-HIGH trial have thrown into question the role of niacin. I don't know the answer. The HATS trial was compelling in study design and outcome; the AIM-HIGH trial also had good design and interpretation. Where does that leave niacin?

LASTLY, there is the possibility that the results may not be reliable. There is a small chance that research, even from reputable institutions, may be under a cloud of suspicion. In 2010 it was discovered that an oncological researcher had manipulated the data in a number of his widely distributed papers to prove that a theory worked[8]. He was considered by many as being at the forefront of ovarian cancer research. He was based at the Duke University, considered an eminent medical institution[9]. This is one of the most significant cases in recent times[10]. However, there are more and no one knows how much impropriety is not detected. Where do vested interests intersect with funding proposals, publishing demands and a genuine and hopeful optimism to prove a truth, regardless of the results?

So, knowledge gaps, or evidence-free zones, have always and will always exist. It just is not possible to answer every question with every variable and then have the situation in which that can be applied to every individual, based on an averaged result that has been demonstrated in a population – assuming that is, that the right study was undertaken, with the right conduct.

Good medicine

In many ways, this represents the art of medicine and the reason why doctors will continue to exist, in spite of improving access to technology and information. **The role of an experienced medical practitioner is to evaluate the individual and that person's particular needs and then, knowing and being familiar with the evidence base and experience in other individuals, come to a conclusion which leads to an appropriate management plan**[1].

I try to explain this to my patients in a way that paints doctors a little like astronomers.

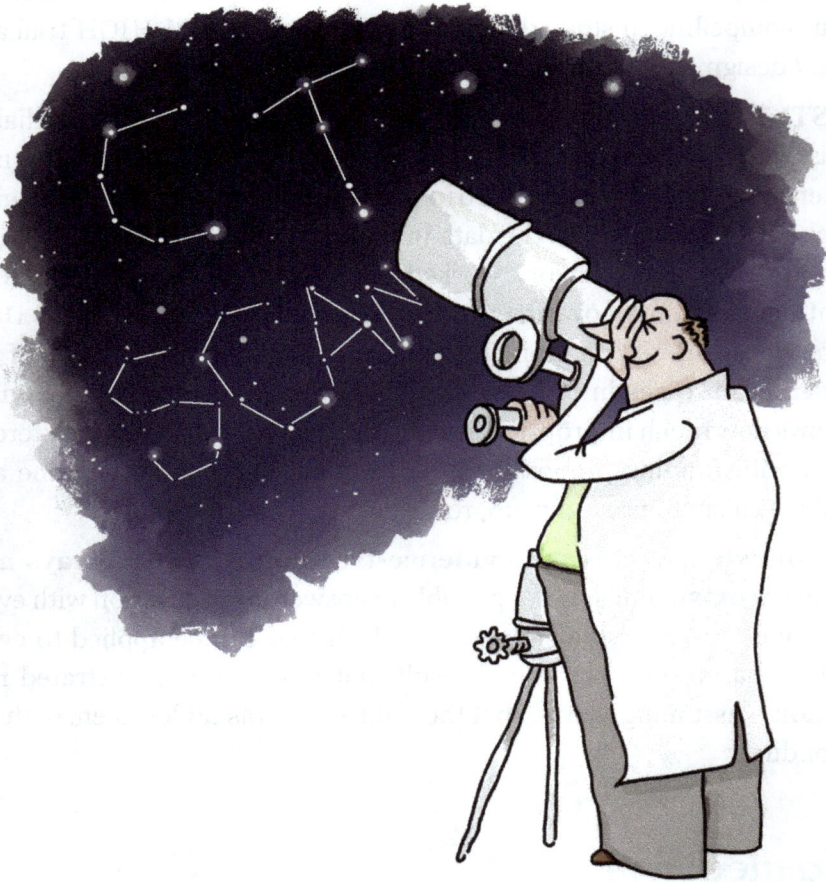

We look out into a universe that we do not fully understand, nor do we fully know its boundaries. Within that universe there are constellations, stars and moons. These are fixed points within that vast space that we have some certainty about. In medicine the fixed points are studies, trials that provide the 'evidence base'. When faced with an individual patient, it is our role to try to most appropriately fit our knowledge of that universe of information to the individual. It may be for a certain patient that we align those stars of knowledge into Orion. For another patient, we may rearrange those stars of knowledge to a different constellation, perhaps Capricorn or Aquarius, or the Big Dipper.

Being aware of where the evidence base lies is absolutely critical in appropriate care. It is also absolutely critical to be aware that the application of that evidence base has limitations and boundaries. It is our role to understand those boundaries as well as our patients and, through experience, try to find the best solution, the best answers and the best care for them.

Accepting their significance but, for the moment, putting aside the lack of evidence-based trials, what if we could identify patients who were going to have a heart attack soon and start primary prevention therapy before they have their coronary event?

This would require us to be far more precise in our evaluation of the **individual** and far less reliant on the risk of that individual within a **population.** What if in an intermediate-risk population, a group in which 15 people out of 100 will have an event in a 10 year period, we were able to find those 15 and start primary prevention therapy before their events?

While no formal, randomised study like this has been done (so it is an evidence-free zone) I put to you that, logically, it would seem that, if we can improve the way we find those high-risk people within the intermediate-risk population, then there is every chance we can make a meaningful difference.

IMPORTANT POINTS ✓

- Current medical practice is founded on the concept of evidence-based medicine. This is the appropriate way to advance medical knowledge.

- However, sole reliance on this approach presents limitations, including:

  » the enormous complexities in medical/biological systems;

  » an individual patient may be different from the averaged population;

  » not all studies can be done, ethically and morally;

  » a study may be inadequately designed;

  » studies can appear to provide conflicting information, and

  » not all results are reliable.

- Medicine is like the universe: it is not fully understood nor are its boundaries accurately known. This leaves room for the 'art of medicine'.

[1]   Sackett DL, Rosenberg WMC, Gray JAM, Haynes RB, Richardson WS. Evidence based medicine: what it is and what it isn't. BMJ 1996;312:71-72.

[2]   Fang J, George MG, Gindi RM, et al. Use of low-dose aspirin as secondary prevention of atherosclerotic cardiovascular disease in US adults (from the National Health Interview Survey, 2012). The American Journal of Cardiology 2015;115:895-900.

[3]   Collaborative meta-analysis of randomised trials of antiplatelet therapy for prevention of death, myocardial infarction, and stroke in high-risk patients. BMJ 2002;324:71-86.

[4]   Smith GCS, Pell JP. Parachute use to prevent death and major trauma related to gravitational challenge: systematic review of randomised controlled trials. BMJ (Clinical research ed) 2003;327:1459-61.

[5]   Arad Y, Spadaro LA, Roth M, Newstein D, Guerci AD. Treatment of asymptomatic adults with elevated coronary calcium scores with atorvastatin, vitamin C, and vitamin E: the St. Francis Heart Study randomized clinical trial. J Am Coll Cardiol 2005;46:166-72.

[6]   Brown BG, Zhao XQ, Chait A, et al. Simvastatin and niacin, antioxidant vitamins, or the combination for the prevention of coronary disease. The New England journal of medicine 2001;345:1583-92.

[7]   Investigators A-H, Boden WE, Probstfield JL, et al. Niacin in patients with low HDL cholesterol levels receiving intensive statin therapy. The New England journal of medicine 2011;365:2255-67.

[8]   Rothschild D, Biggest Offender of Medical Research Misconduct in History? 2012. Feb 16, 2012 4:11:00 PM (Accessed at http://www.ithenticate.com/plagiarism-detection-blog/bid/78874 Biggest-Offender-of-Medical-Research-Misconduct-in-History#.Vo5a9_l95hF.)

[9]   Pelley S, Deception at Duke. CBS News, 2012. February 12th, 2012 (Accessed at http://www.cbsnews.com/8301-18560_162-57376073/deception-at-duke/.)

[10] Oransky I, The Anil Potti retraction record so far. Retraction Watch, 2012. February 14th, 2012 (Accessed at http://retractionwatch.wordpress.com/2012/02/14 the-anil-potti-retraction-record-so-far/.)

In the next chapter we consider new possibilities for preventative cardiology.

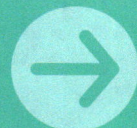

A personal approach to managing the individual rather than the population in an attempt to stop a heart attack before it occurs

The remainder of the book reflects my approach to primary prevention of coronary artery disease or stopping a heart attack before it occurs. I offer it to you in an effort to bring as much information as possible to the appropriate management of an individual, understanding the lack of a clear-cut evidence base but drawing from observational data, common sense and the 'art of medicine'.

Dr Warrick Bishop is an experienced cardiologist with extensive training and expertise in the area of CT coronary angiography. His very proactive approach to cardiac health has been an integral part of his methodology throughout his career. Having known Warrick for 25 years, I can assure you it is not a recent fashionable trend. His practice has always been and remains very focussed on 'best care' for individual cardiac patients as he takes a holistic approach to patient management.

Alistair Begg, cardiologist, Adelaide

Chapter 5 -
Image is everything

IN THIS CHAPTER WE LOOK AT

> medical and technological advances that make possible new opportunities for primary preventative cardiology

A key element to any new approach to primary prevention and risk assessment is the availability of, and accessibility to, imaging the coronary arteries using CT scanning. This is a non-invasive, safe way to evaluate the build-up of cholesterol, or atheroma, to give an indication of the health of the coronary arteries in an asymptomatic person. Central to this, we must understand that a build-up of cholesterol within the arteries generally leads to **associated deposits of calcium** in the artery, so that calcium can be used as an indicator of plaque build-up.

Calcium

For more than 80 years, observations have been made, primarily by radiologists in the earlier years, that calcium could build up in the arteries, although there were differing opinions about its significance.

As far back as 1930 observations were made by German physician R. Lenk[1] in an article, "Rontgendiagnose der koronarsklerose in vivo", that calcium could be detected in the coronary arteries of "living subjects". This was reported again in 1959 in the United States by D. H. Blankenhorn and D. Stearne[2] who, using x-rays on cadavers, demonstrated the presence of calcification within the coronary arteries. About the same time, in the United Kingdom, M. F. Oliver and his colleagues[3] used fluoroscopy (or rapid acquisition x-ray to allow assessment during movement) to assess coronary artery disease using calcium as an indicator of potential problems in living subjects.

A study by McGuire in 1968[4] looked at calcification within the coronary arteries in patients who had had symptoms of angina or who had had a heart attack compared with a control group who had had no known problems. This simple study, which evaluated several hundred people, suggested that the development of calcification within the coronary arteries may be a useful guide or indicator of risk in an individual. The summary from that study is:

Five hundred and forty-four unselected patients were examined by a radiologist to determine the presence or absence of coronary artery calcification. The overall incidence of coronary calcification was 20 percent and there was a definite increase in the frequency of the finding with increasing age. A comparison of 94 patients with coronary calcification with a matched control group, without calcification, indicated that the prevalence of symptomatic ischaemic heart disease in the group with calcification was approximately twice that of the control group. The correlation was even more significant when the degree of calcification was moderate or severe. (Ischaemic heart disease is reduced blood supply to the heart.)

No Calcification

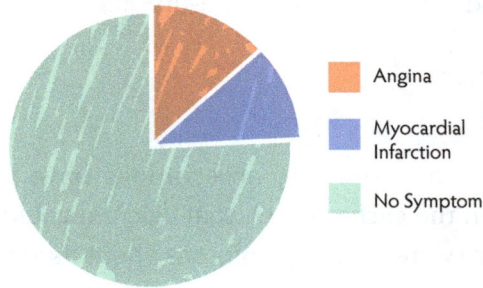

- Angina
- Myocardial Infarction
- No Symptom

Calcification Present

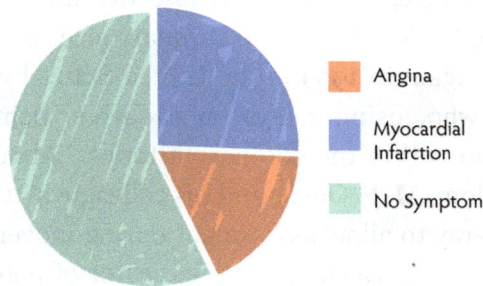

- Angina
- Myocardial Infarction
- No Symptom

The McGuire study shows that the more green, the better. It is easy to see that the presence of calcification is associated with less green.

Although this observational study was undertaken almost 50 years ago, it is engaging in terms of suggesting the possibility that imaging of the coronary arteries could be a valuable indicator of the risk an individual patient carries. Although this early work was interesting and potentially tantalising in the opportunities it offered, it was not really picked up. This is probably because the process used high amounts of x-ray radiation, was limited by the availability of fluoroscopy and offered limited quantification of the findings, which were described as "not present", "mild", "moderate" or "severe".

It was not until the 1980s when a technology called **electron beam computed tomography** (EBCT) became available that interest was again ignited in trying to evaluate the health of an individual's coronary arteries. EBCT simply means that, using enormous magnets, x-rays are deflected at very high speed to acquire images which are then reconstructed, giving rise to the term **computed tomography** (CT). In the 1980s EBCT scanners were large and extremely expensive and only a few machines existed worldwide.

It is important to understand that imaging the heart has always been difficult because the heart moves and so any method of imaging needs to be extremely fast.

An American cardiologist, Arthur Agatston, realised a potential value in imaging or scanning the heart arteries to make an assessment of the amount of calcium within them, to potentially aid in risk assessment. Agatston published his work in 1990 and the **Agatston Score** has become a standardised method of evaluating the coronary arteries for the presence of calcification[5]. The score uses three millimetre slices (defined by the EBCT specifications) through the heart and then a combination of volume and density of the calcium detected to generate a number or 'score'.

In 1996, a pathologist, J. A. Rumberger, established the clear relationship between calcium and cholesterol within the structure of atheromatous plaque. Rumberger showed that **calcium moved into the wall of the artery following the deposition of cholesterol and then scavenger cells, with subsequent formation of scar tissue within a plaque**[6].

This is an important point that I make to my patients. Calcium acts as a *marker* of the process with which we are concerned, that is, the presence of atherosclerotic plaque within the arteries.

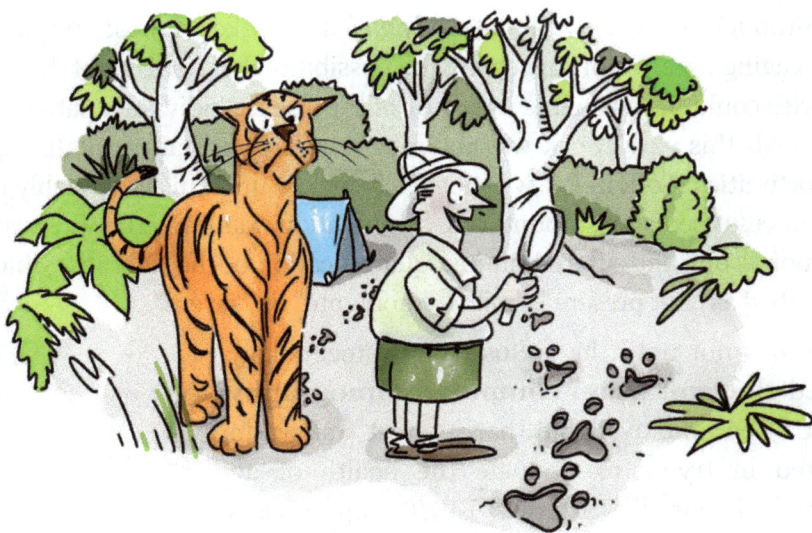

Calcium is the tiger's footprint and atheroma is the tiger.

Often patients will ask, "What can we do to get rid of the calcium?" but calcium is not the issue. **Calcium is simply the surrogate marker we use to give an indication of the process we are concerned about, the build-up of plaque within the coronary arteries.** I use the example that if, on pitching a tent in the jungle, we saw lots of tiger foot prints, it would mean that tigers are around and it might not be a great place to pitch the tent. Not seeing tiger foot prints doesn't mean there are not tigers in the area but it certainly makes it a better place to pitch a tent.

The calcium is a bystander, not the problem. Calcium itself is fairly inert in arteries, so it can stay there. We are wanting to deal with the process that put it there.

Supplements

Patients often are already taking a calcium supplement and/or vitamin D, and are concerned about whether or not they should continue. The jury is still out on this[7].

There is inconclusive data in relation to supplementation and coronary calcification. My general recommendation, however, is that if there are significant issues with the bones (osteoporosis or 'thin bones') such that supplementation is indicated, then supplementation should be considered.

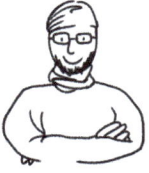

If there are no clear issues with the bones I suggest that vitamin D is probably best taken by sun exposure to the skin. There is no naturally occurring oral form of vitamin D (and remember, some oral dosages can lead to levels far higher than seen physiologically). Similarly, I suggest dietary calcium (cheese, dairy, meat, yoghurt) is also the most natural way. By virtue of the amount of calcium contained in them, taking tablets will lead to levels of calcium in the bloodstream that are far greater than would be seen in nature. This is best avoided, I suggest, until we know more about it.

CT technology evolution

CT technology has moved on a long way since the 1980s and 90s. Since about 2006, a new generation of CT machines has become available. These machines are smaller, faster, cheaper and use the same or less radiation than the original EBCT scanners.

Today's CT scanners image the heart using a gantry system (a large ring) that spins x-ray heads and detectors around the patient at high speed. Each rotation of image acquisition can obtain from four centimetres to the full vertical distance of the heart. The speed of rotation is very fast, and continues to increase with improvements in technology. Because the heart is constantly moving, the faster the image can be acquired, the less blur and the better quality of the image. This is similar to using fast shutter speeds on regular cameras to take action photographs. These new machines, with more detectors and faster rotation times, are being used with advanced technologies that reduce the radiation doses to below ordinary yearly background radiation.

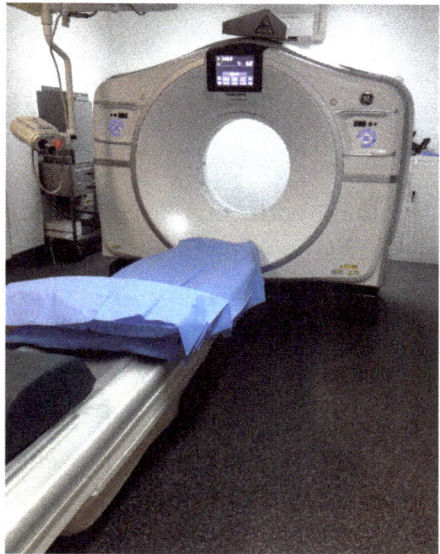

This means that our current technology is able to **accurately, reliably** and **reproducibly** acquire images of the arteries of the heart for evaluation of calcification. The current generation of machines is validated to apply the score generated by Agatston et al[8].

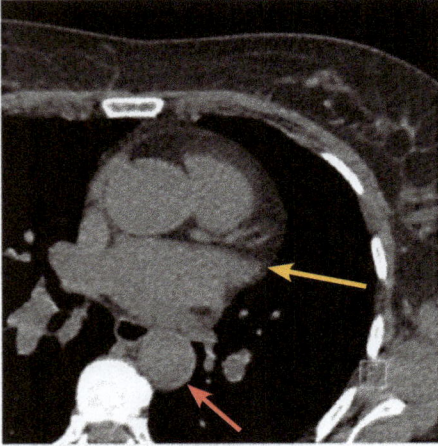

This is an image of zero calcium score. The yellow arrow points to the heart; the red arrow to the aorta.

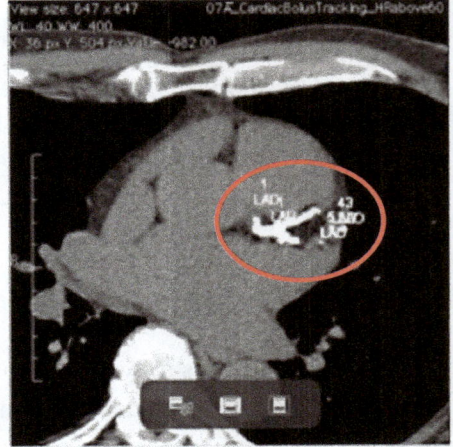

This is an image showing extensive calcification of the left anterior descending artery and circumflex artery.

Along with increased speed, improved image acquisition and the reduction of the radiation dose, there has been increasing interest in injecting contrast into the vein in a patient's arm and then tracking that contrast through the body, into the arteries of the heart, to then outline the arteries. This is called a **coronary computed tomography angiogram** or a CCTA, often referred to as a CT coronary angiogram.

Further to showing the presence of calcium, **CT coronary angiography outlines the coronary artery in exquisite detail**, giving information about the location of plaque, the quality and nature of the plaque, degree of stenosis and size of vessel affected. **This information had previously not been obtainable, non-invasively, in a living patient.**

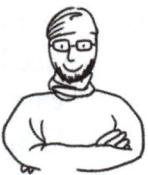

The development of this technology, together with the development of protocols for imaging, both of calcium within the arteries and tracing contrast through the arteries to outline specific detail, are major changes in what is available when assessing the coronary arteries

and a patient's risk potential. This combined imaging of coronary calcium scoring and CT coronary angiography provides an opportunity to make an evaluation of an individual patient's arteries and the patient's individual risk, as opposed to what the risk may be in a population of patients with similar risk factors.

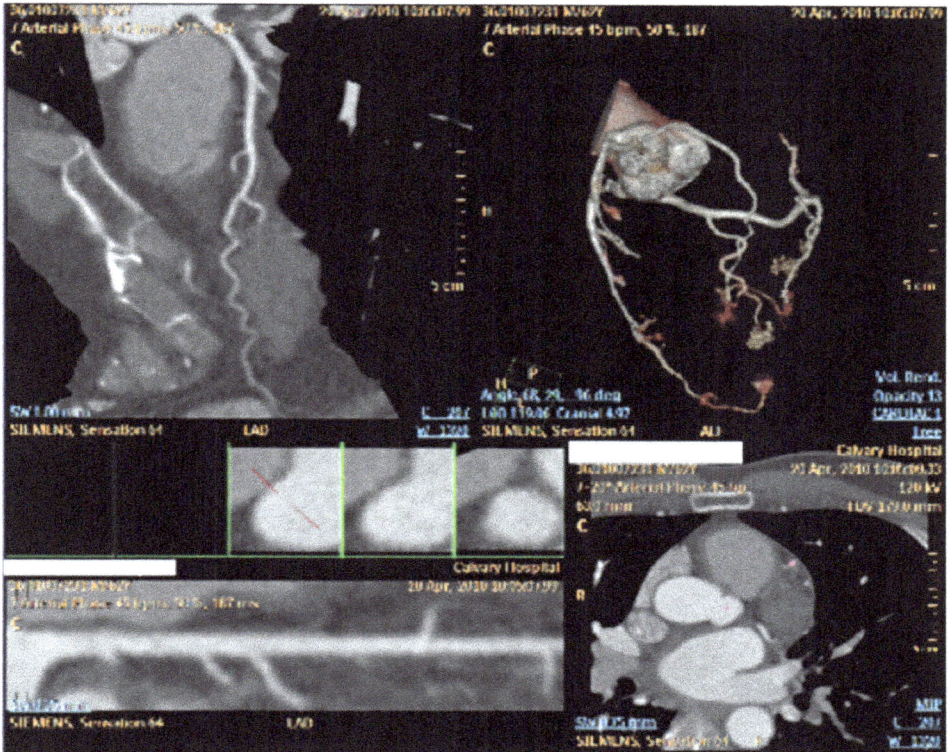

This image shows the amazing detail of a CT coronary angiogram. This is the information available to the doctor reviewing or reporting a CCTA on a specially dedicated workstation.

The top left is the artery isolated within the other chest structures.
The top right is the 3D reconstruction of the patient's coronary tree.
The bottom right is the horizontal slices through the chest, also called axials.
The bottom left is called a spindle view and is the artery stretched out straight and can be spun on its axis.
These images are too complex to cover in this discussion but you can appreciate the fantastic pictures we can see.

IMPORTANT POINTS ✓

- Calcium has been observed in the arteries of living subjects for more than 80 years. Over time this has become standardised with the use of the Agatston Score during non-contrast CT imaging.

- More recently, technology has improved and now dye/contrast can be injected during a CT scan to outline the coronary arteries in exquisite detail.

- Combining non-contrast and contrast CT imaging of the heart gives previously unobtainable information about the coronary arteries that can add to the risk assessment of an individual.

[1]   Lenk R. Rontgendiagnose der Koronarsklerose in vivo. Fortschr ad Geb d 1927.

[2]   Blankenhorn DH, Stern D. Calcification of the coronary arteries. Am J Roentgenol Radium Ther Nucl Med 1959;81:772-7.

[3]   Oliver MF, Samuel E, Morley P, Young GB, Kapur PL. Detection of Coronary-Artery Calcification during Life. Lancet 1964;1:891-5.

[4]   McGuire J, Chou TC, Schneider HJ. Visualization of calcification of the coronary arteries by the image intensifier. Transactions of the American Clinical and Climatological Association 1968;79:61-66.

[5]   Agatston AS, Janowitz WR, Hildner FJ, Zusmer NR, Viamonte M, Jr., Detrano R. Quantification of coronary artery calcium using ultrafast computed tomography. J Am Coll Cardiol 1990;15:827-32.

[6]   Wexler L, Brundage B, Crouse J, et al. Coronary Artery Calcification: Pathophysiology, Epidemiology, Imaging Methods, and Clinical Implications: A Statement for Health Professionals From the American Heart Association. Circulation 1996;94:1175-92.

[7]   Manson JE, Allison MA, Carr JJ, et al. Calcium/vitamin D supplementation and coronary artery calcification. Menopause (New York, NY) 2010;17:683.

[8]   Schmermund A, Erbel R, Silber S. Age and gender distribution of coronary artery calcium measured by four-slice computed tomography in 2,030 persons with no symptoms of coronary artery disease. American Journal of Cardiology;90:168-73.

Cardiac CT imaging's ability to evaluate the extent of cholesterol build-up before the onset of a problem is discussed more fully in the next chapter. →

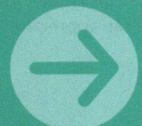

Chapter 6 -
Changing times, changing terminology

IN THIS CHAPTER WE LOOK AT 👁

> what is a disease before it is a disease?
  coronary atheroma burden

> risk factors vs localised findings

The ability for cardiac CT imaging to demonstrate the presence of atheroma or plaque within the arteries is a paradigm shift in the conventional management of coronary artery disease.

As discussed earlier, historically, coronary artery disease has been diagnosed at the time of the event, the time a patient has had chest pain, shortness of breath or a major adverse coronary event. By that time, the patient has developed a 'disease' which simply means a symptom or loss of normal function.

Changing terminology

I have patients who undergo cardiac CT imaging for risk evaluation and in whom we demonstrate the presence of plaque build-up. These are otherwise healthy patients looking to maximise their primary prevention strategies. **This is the exciting opportunity that cardiac CT imaging offers; it gives us an ability to evaluate the extent of plaque build-up *before* the onset of a problem.** Intuitively, one might think this is extremely valuable in the process of attempting to evaluate the potential risk that an individual may carry in regard to the development of coronary artery disease. Yet, although cardiac CT imaging has been readily available for the past 5 to 10 years, there has been no clear consensus for the description of plaque formation prior to the occurrence of symptoms or loss of function, to describe the 'pre-disease state'.

In these cases, I do not feel comfortable calling formation of plaque in the arteries 'coronary artery disease' before an event or problem, and in a patient without any symptoms. There are four reasons why I specifically avoid the term 'disease' in describing plaque formation found on scanning **before** a patient has had any problems.

1. *It is not yet a disease.* As the patient has not experienced any event or symptom, the term 'disease' is not well received by the patient. It is much easier to have the conversation around a "build-up of cholesterol in the arteries that needs management", than label the patient as having a 'disease'. There is significant psychological cost in diagnosing a 'disease' particularly in a patient who has presented in a primary preventive capacity, and is otherwise feeling well. My objective, as a preventative cardiologist, is to keep that patient healthy and well, with the goal being to avoid the development of 'disease'.

2. *Coronary artery disease, as a term, has no variation or scope of degree that can be applied to it.* It is binary; it is either present or not. If we are looking at someone who has a build-up of plaque in the arteries, it could be severe, minimal or somewhere in between. This subtlety or gradation of severity is not conveyed in the term 'coronary artery disease'.

3. *Cholesterol deposition within the arteries appears to be part of the ageing process.* If any of us were to live long enough we would all have evidence of wear and tear within our coronary arteries. The final common result of this would be the development of atheromatous plaque. That this occurs more rapidly in some people simply reflects individual predisposition and does not necessarily reflect the early stages of a 'disease state'. If we accept ageing as a natural process and we accept wear and tear as a natural process, then the development of cholesterol deposition and plaque formation within the arteries is on that spectrum. Early in the process, it is simply a predisposition and does not warrant the label 'disease'. A parallel example might be someone who has a 'clicky' hip or a 'clicky' knee which, in many years to come, *may* lead to arthritic change and eventually require the replacement of an arthritic joint. However, in the early stages, it is simply showing signs of wear and tear, or features consistent with ageing.

4. *The label of coronary artery disease has immediate and rigid implications in situations such as insurance or licensing,* situations that may lead to a knee jerk response or reaction without attention to gradation or severity, resulting in a misdirected or disproportionate response.

The term I use with patients and in correspondence in a primary preventative setting, to describe finding plaque within the arteries in a patient who is otherwise well, is **coronary atheroma burden.** This is a description for the **extent of plaque formation within the coronary arteries as demonstrated on imaging before the development of disease.** The use of this terminology then allows more precision around the description of the cardiac CT findings, such that a patient may demonstrate low-risk atheroma burden, high-risk atheroma burden or something in between. *(I explore this concept in more detail Appendix 1.)*

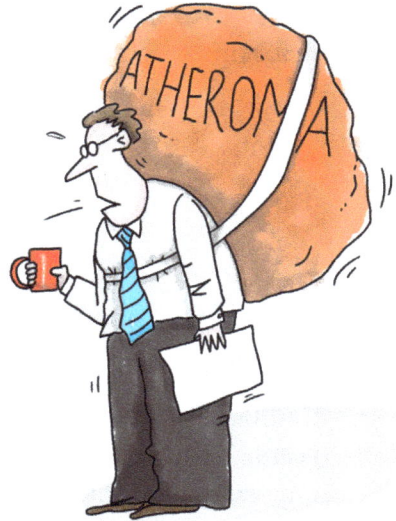

Changing our understanding

The other significant observation is that as we image coronary arteries in a primary prevention role, we are discovering that **the plaque formation can be very localised.** The interesting thing about this is that our risk factor model for the evaluation of the likely development of a problem with coronary artery disease focusses on factors which affect the whole body: age, cholesterol, blood pressure, diabetes, smoking, diet and exercise. One could think these factors would also affect a coronary artery equally – but they do not!

Imaging clearly demonstrates that plaque formation may occur in only one or two locations within the coronary artery tree. This means that an individual's future may be defined by a single plaque that is little more than a centimetre in length. Remembering that the main branches of the coronary arteries are 35-40cm in combined total length, this is a small fraction of the coronary tree, yet it may determine a life or death outcome for the patient.

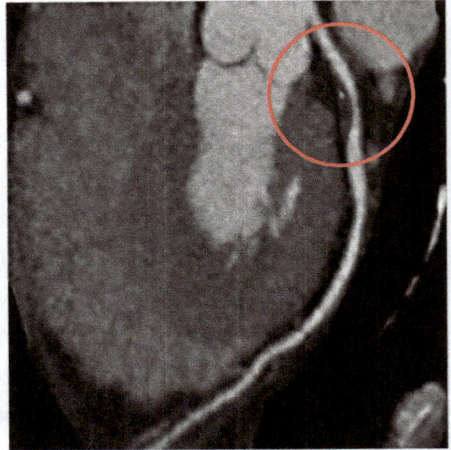

This scan shows one large life-threatening proximal plaque in the left anterior descending artery. The remainder of the LAD and the other vessels in this patient were clear of plaque.

This means that there is an interplay between local factors within the artery and the risk factors which the individual may have:

- traditional risk factors, based on observational studies over many years, clearly indicate that certain cardiovascular risk factors are important associations in the development of coronary artery disease in an individual, and

- there is no question that there are local features within an individual's arteries that may potentially be regulated by these more general risk factors.

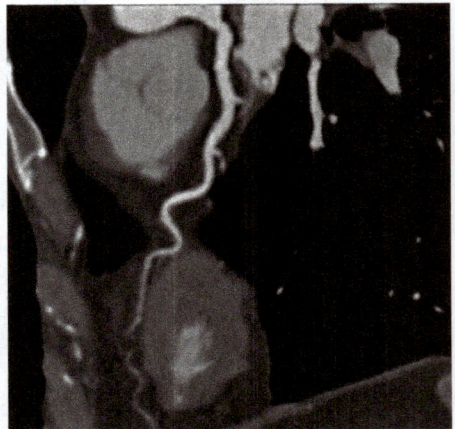

The complexity of this is that there are people who have what would be considered high-level cardiovascular risk factors and yet there are no local features within their arteries and no development of plaque.

HIGH-RISK FACTORS, NO LOCAL FACTORS
This patient was a 62-year-old male with the following lipid profile:
TC 9.1, TG 3.3, HDL 1.5, Ratio 6.6, LDL 6.6.
He had also been non-insulin dependant diabetic for five years.
Surprisingly, there is no evidence of atheroma burden.

Conversely, there may be patients who have low or intermediate cardiovascular risk factors but significant local predisposition in their arteries, showing substantial or high risk atheroma burden.

The only way we can sensibly deal with this situation, in my opinion, is to understand that **our prediction based on risk factors alone is only part of the puzzle.** This may be accurate for dealing with large populations but falls short for the individual when we have no mechanism for assessing local factors within the artery.

It is with this background that the role of imaging the arteries in an individual begins to make more sense.

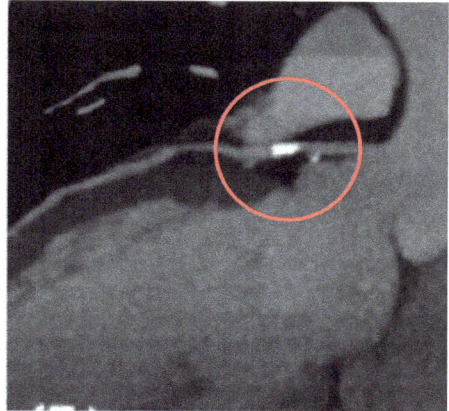

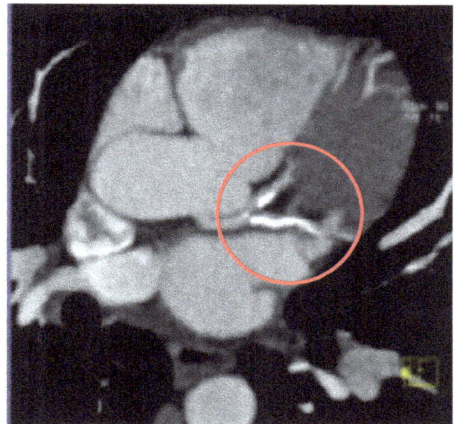

AVERAGE RISK FACTORS, SIGNIFICANT LOCAL FACTORS
This well 48-year-old male had no diabetes and a lipid profile of
TC 5.8, HDL 1.1, TG 1.3 (unremarkable).
He undertook very regular exercise, was not over-weight, had no family history, no hypertension and did not smoke. The scan shows surprisingly extensive atheroma burden.

IMPORTANT POINTS ☑

- Cardiac CT reveals the extent and distribution of plaque in the arteries.

- 'Disease' is defined by symptoms or loss of function.

- 'Coronary artery disease' refers to the complications (symptoms or loss of function) from build-up of cholesterol in the arteries.

- Cholesterol build-up **before** a problem occurs is perhaps best referred to as **atheroma burden** as it has not yet become a 'disease'.

- Plaque burden can be very localised, suggesting that local factors within the artery must also play a role in plaque development.

- Combining non-contrast and contrast cardiac CT imaging of the heart gives previously unobtainable information about the coronary arteries. Atheroma burden can be assessed in relation to its location and before complications arise. This can aid risk assessment and management for the individual.

Common scenarios that present for cardiovascular risk management are highlighted in the next chapter. →

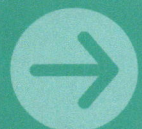

Chapter 7 -
What about my arteries?

> common investigative scenarios

General practitioners (GPs) refer to me to assist in particular situations of cardiovascular risk management for their patients. Due to my belief in the investigative value of the technology and the process, and having been involved in the establishment of a cardiac CT service for the local region, I have developed a particular interest in cardiac CT imaging and related information that help in decisions around future risk and patient management. I have been involved in the assessment, preparation, reading of the study and interpretation of the findings, and then the application of that information to individual patients in close to 3000 cases. The most common scenarios I deal with are patients who don't want to take statins or they are intolerant of them, there is a family history of heart problems or they want reassurance.

"I don't want to take statins"

I often see patients with high risk factors who do not want to take statins, drugs that can lower cholesterol in the blood. In recent years there has been significant media interest and comment surrounding the role of statins, causing confusion and

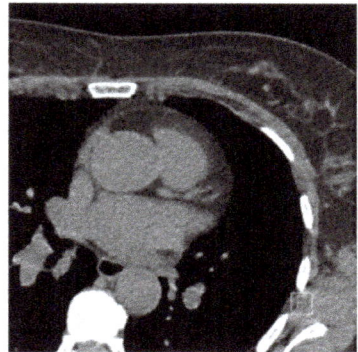

This is a zero calcium score in a 66-year-old active female who had worked hard on lifestyle modification for three years as she wanted to avoid statin therapy. She had a total cholesterol of 8.8, triglyceride of 1.3, a high density lipoprotein of 2.0 and a low density lipoprotein of 6.6 with a ratio of 4.4. Fasting glucose was 5.1 and she had been started on 20mg of rosuvastatin (a statin) by her GP. With a zero score, the literature suggests that her risk of a MACE in the next 10 years is less than one percent. This is the case, even with her high cholesterol levels.

uncertainty concerning their benefits, as well as raising questions about possible side-effects. There are many patients who have been started on cholesterol-lowering agents by their GP, in the context of cardiovascular risk, but who would rather not be on a medication, unless that medication were absolutely necessary.

Intolerant of statins

I also see patients with high cholesterol levels and high-risk features but who are intolerant of statins. Both patients and GPs manifest a sense of frustration as there is difficulty in achieving appropriate cholesterol targets in an individual who, with elevated cholesterol and a perceived high risk, is intolerant of the agent. The reason for the referral to me is for an evaluation to produce extra information that could provide more guidance in terms of the individual's needs.

The questions being asked are: *What is going on in the arteries? Is this patient's risk really as high as imagined? Is there evidence of significant plaque build-up in the arteries? Does this patient need to persist with the statins and be more accepting of (mild to moderate) side-effects? Could this patient be managed on a lower dose of statin? Is this patient's risk likely to be low, given there is minimal or no clear evidence of coronary cholesterol build-up? Perhaps the perceived risk, which is a population-based risk, is not accurate for this individual?*

I discuss the balance between traditional risk factor prediction and the cardiac CT risk in a user guide for doctors in Appendix 3.

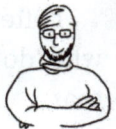

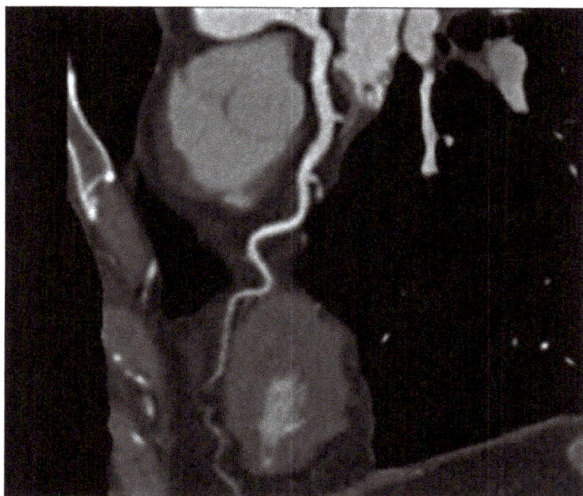

This is a cardiac CT image of a 62-year-old male who is statin intolerant. His total cholesterol was 9.1, his triglyceride was 3.3, his high density lipoprotein was 1.5, his low density lipoprotein was 6.6 and his total cholesterol to HDL ratio was 6.6. He had been a non-insulin dependent diabetic for five years. He had tried every statin given at high doses because of his cholesterol level and each had given him liver abnormality. He was a non-smoker, with normal blood pressure and no family history of premature coronary artery disease. He had no symptoms. The cardiac CT showed negligible or very low-risk atheroma build-up.

This patient's risk factors cannot be ignored. However, the finding of low-risk features (almost nothing!) in his arteries means that, at least in the short to intermediate term, his risks are much lower than predicted from risk calculation. This may then allow the introduction of a statin at lower doses, in an effort to avoid the liver side-effects, and an acceptance that treating to strict targets may not be immediately critical.

Family history of heart problems

I see numerous patients who have a significant family history of premature coronary artery disease (male younger than 55 years old or female younger than 60 years old who has had a MACE) but who seem to have relatively low- or intermediate-risk features, based on standard cardiovascular risk calculation. These patients come, knowing that there has been the loss of family members at a young age, unexpectedly and, understandably, very traumatically. These patients, quite reasonably, want to know if they are at the same risk. It is often the case that standard cardiovascular risk calculators do not include family history as one of the variables and so, young patients, particularly with concerning family histories, are often poorly risk-categorised by standard risk calculators.

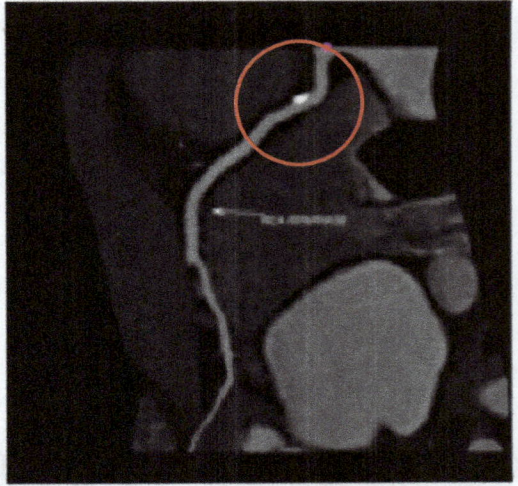

This is the cardiac CT of a 42-year-old male whose father died aged 51 and whose grandfather died at 53. The man's lipid profile was completely unremarkable, with a total cholesterol to high density lipoprotein ratio of 4 and normal triglycerides. He played competitive sport and was a smoker. The cardiac CT clearly shows early plaque formation at the beginning of the right coronary artery. After the scan, the patient started appropriate risk management therapy and quit smoking.

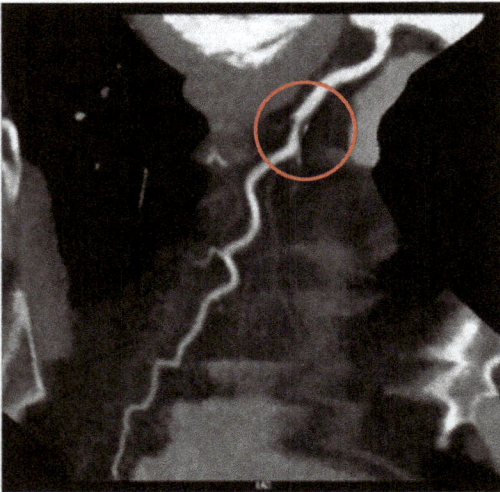

This is the CT angiogram of a 65-year-old exploration geologist with an untidy lipid profile and a lifestyle not conducive to good healthy habits. Travelling to places like the Congo, Peru and outback Australia, he wanted to know if he was going to have a heart attack in some remote far-flung region of the world. With these findings of high-risk plaque in the LAD, we were able to implement therapy to reduce his risk of event and increase the chance of his returning home safely after his trips away.

"I just want to know"

The final group consists of those in the low- to intermediate-risk group who simply want some clarity for themselves around risk. They may have borderline blood pressure, carry a little extra weight, exhibit borderline cholesterol levels, don't exercise as much as they think they should. However, they have seen friends, colleagues or loved ones who were seemingly well and not obviously at increased risk, have coronary events or die. These people are seeking some clarity and certainty around their personal risk, rather than the risk that may be attributable to a population with similar characteristics.

IMPORTANT POINTS

- Common scenarios point to the complexities and variations that build further support for the premise that knowing the individual's **actual** situation is greatly preferable for treatment, management and reassurance than relying on population-based averages.

Let's have a sensible discussion about statins before moving on to a more detailed look at the role of calcium as an indicator of potential risk.

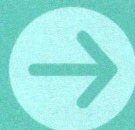

why all the fuss about statins?

These days I spend a considerable amount of time speaking with patients about the pros and cons of statin therapy, as in recent times there has been increasing discussion around the negative effects of these agents. Some commentators suggest that a high cholesterol reading does not mean a patient should immediately take a statin, as not all patients with raised cholesterol will develop coronary artery disease. I agree with this; throughout the book I discuss how looking at the coronary arteries can help us determine who really is at high risk and who isn't.

I prefer to reframe the discussion around the role of statins. I think it is more sensible to recognise that each medication, including statins, has risks. The question then becomes: **what are the benefits to the patient?** Before we get into that, however, what is a statin?

What is a statin?

A statin is a group of drugs used to lower cholesterol. The statin works by blocking an enzyme in the liver called HMG-CoA reductase.   There are several statins available: simvastatin, atorvastatin, pravastatin, fluvastatin and rosuvastatin. Each agent has a different potency and some difference in chemical qualities. As an example, atorvastatin is 'lipophillic', meaning that it moves into fatty tissue, while rosuvastatin is 'lipophobic', meaning that it doesn't move into fatty tissue.

Each statin acts to lower available cholesterol in the liver, leading to a reduction primarily of LDL cholesterol in the serum. Cholesterol, however, is not all bad. It is also important in synthesis of hormones, particularly the mineralocorticoids, which have a role in regulating fluid balance and blood

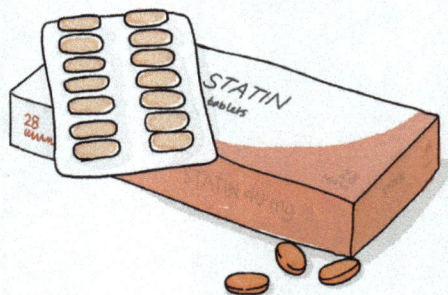

pressure, the glucocorticoids which are the steroids involved in immune response, and also the sex hormones.

The internet means everyone can consult 'Dr Google' and so patients come to me 'well informed' and with 'a plan', and often many with questions and concerns: "I want to manage my cholesterol with diet and exercise"; "What about the effect on memory?"; "What about the effect on hormones?"; "I don't want to take a tablet unless I have to"; "I've tried a statin before and it didn't agree with me".

I believe the basis for discussion is fairly clear-cut and, in fact, is how we should deal with any intervention: **We discuss the *risks* of the medication versus the *benefits* that the individual will gain from taking the medication.** If a patient has high cholesterol and no evidence of plaque build-up in the arteries, then taking a statin is (side-effect) risk-**without**-benefit. This is a situation when it is hard to justify the patient taking the medication. The flip side also holds. If the arteries show significant build-up of plaque, then taking a statin is (side-effect) risk-**with**-benefit, when taking the medication makes sense.

The statin and cholesterol story

The statin story began around 25 years ago with the publication of the 4S study[1] that suggested this new class of agent had an effect in reducing MACE. This opened a floodgate of drug companies trying to develop their own compound and demonstrate its benefit in large multicentre, randomised double-blind trials, the sort of trials that were to become the foundation blocks of 'evidence-based' medicine.

This focus on lowering cholesterol then reframed the way we collectively viewed cholesterol as a risk factor. It became, and has remained, the situation that **we think of high cholesterol as relating to high risk of heart disease. THIS IS NOT ALWAYS THE CASE** *and I discuss this throughout this book, explaining the difference between association and causation.*

The important point to understand in the cholesterol story is that to use blood cholesterol levels to predict if someone is at risk of heart disease can be inaccurate in the individual. However, if we find that an individual has coronary artery disease or high-risk atheroma burden, then the literature suggests that treating those individuals with a statin will reduce their risk of an event.

With the widespread availability of statins and a misdirected belief that cholesterol is the problem, many patients have been put on cholesterol-lowering medication in a primary prevention situation when they may have no build-up of cholesterol in the arteries and no plaque, and so will take a medication with its possible side-effects and see no beneficial outcome: **all risk** and **no benefit!**

This is when cardiac CT imaging can provide critical information regarding the *individual's* coronary arteries to *clarify* risk *and* benefit. When we know the health of an individual's arteries, we can then be clear about the benefit that person will obtain from taking a statin (or not) with its risk of side-effects.

Side-effects

The side-effects of statins are well documented. Statins are without doubt, collectively, the most studied and most prescribed medication in human history.

Well, what are the side-effects?

When asked, I often say that the side-effect we are hoping for is longevity. Jokes aside though, I have to say that, as a general rule, I don't tell patients what side-effects may arise from a medication, not to be paternalistic but rather I'm aware of the power of suggestion and placebo. I have learnt over the years that, if I forewarn a patient that a medication may cause slight dizziness or blurred vision, 50 percent of patients will have dizziness or blurred vision before they leave my office! These days, helpful pharmacists also provide patients with pages of literature covering side-effects. Conceptually, this is a good idea in terms of education. However, I have these pages given back to me covered with highlighter pen indicting every side-effect the patient has had.

I'm not being dismissive of side-effects. It is absolutely critical to be aware of tolerability, particularly when the patient may be on the medication long term. Yet, I see little point running a 50 percent chance of evoking a placebo effect. What I say to patients is that some people will be allergic and this is completely unpredictable, like reacting to peanut butter. Some patients may have trouble but only a trial of the medication will let us know this. The vast majority of people take them without a problem. After all that is why the drugs have been evaluated by the Therapeutic Goods Administration and we are allowed to prescribe them.

Having said all that, the most common side-effect is muscle aches and pains. Very rarely, this can be severe and is called rhabdomyolysis. This severe reaction is seen about once for every 65,000 patients on a statin. Remember, we are treating a condition that kills approximately one in two people.

Even the development of muscle aches and pains is variable and will be patient specific. As we are giving these agents to patients who are mostly over 50 years of age, separating aches and pains caused by a medication from getting a bit older and stiffer is difficult. I suspect statins are occasionally blamed when ageing, arthritis and a busy day in the garden may be closer to the cause.

Several other concerns are raised occasionally.

• *Statins cause Alzheimer's disease[2].*

This is a complex and concerning claim. I have met patients who swear the statins cause memory impairment in them, yet the vast majority of my patients describe no such symptom. I'm not able to advise if using a different statin alleviates this or not, although it would be the first thing I would try for a patient who clearly would benefit from being on the medication.

Its consideration is also confounded by a condition called vascular dementia caused by multiple small strokes affecting the brain, which could be wrongly attributed to statin use. Yet, statins and aspirin, with good blood pressure control, are part of the recommended therapy. This is another example of when risk of medication versus benefit to the patient would be used as a guide to the decision-making.

• *Statins have an effect on hormones, particularly the sex hormones[3-5].*

This is theoretically possible but difficult to sort out and should be considered on an individual basis.

- *Statins may increase the likelihood of progression to diabetes[6].*

It is important to be aware of, and deal with, this within the context of the individual. Generally, diabetes would be considered the lesser of the two evils if compared with cardiovascular risk in a high-risk individual.

- *Statins cause cancer[7], liver damage, muscle damage (and anything else you can think of).*

I have had every side-effect known to man described to me over the years and anything is possible, as each person is different and will respond in his/her own unique way. For any individual, my effort lies in understanding the benefit the patient will obtain from the medication and then finding a balance between the side-effect (risk from the medication) and the maximal tolerated dose of the best tolerated of the statins. I would only persist with trying to find an acceptable agent and dose if it were clear the patient would benefit from the medication.

What remains most important is being clear about the **risk** and **benefit.**

- If the patient has low-risk atheroma burden, then persisting with a medication with side-effects makes little sense.

- If the patient has known coronary artery disease or a high- to very high-risk atheroma burden, then it is important to find a solution. This patient **will benefit** from the medication and the side-effects need to be managed. In this situation, there are a number of options:

  » Most importantly, be clear it is the statin that is causing the side-effect. This should be evaluated under medical supervision and will require withdrawal of the medication and re-challenge. This may even need to be repeated to be sure.

  » The next thing to try is an alternate agent. Some of the statins are lipid soluble and some are lipophobic. It is worth changing from one to the other to see if this makes a difference.

  » Another thing to try is to lower the dose to a level that doesn't cause side-effects. Doctor and patient need to work closely adjusting (titrating) the dose of the best tolerated statin to find a dose that suits the individual. In my own practice I have some patients on half a tablet of the lowest dose of a statin that they take twice a week without problems. Any more and side-effects impact on their daily well-being. In this situation, a little is better than none at all. There is also the opportunity to use non-statin cholesterol lowering drugs that can work synergistically with the statin to help in management.

Effectiveness?

What I've described is based on **the premise that the statins are beneficial.** Well, some of the controversy is because there is some questioning of their effectiveness.

A number of the early trials have been under the spotlight with questions as to their scientific rigour[8]. There is also the suggestion that statin trials post-2005 are variable in their findings, with not all demonstrating benefit[9]. It becomes very complex to assess as different studies have different populations and end points. This, together with the positive findings of the early statin trials, make it unethical to run a study that denies an at-risk population the best available treatment, thus making the statistically-significant separation of outcomes more difficult.

I don't wish to dwell on the scientific controversy too much other than to say that statistics and graphs can be presented any way you wish to support almost any premise you wish to advance.

What I will say though, is that in my own observation over the past 20 years, I have seen a change in the landscape of coronary artery disease and its presentation. There appears to be an observable improvement in the stability of the patients demonstrated to have coronary artery disease. These patients, who after their first presentation are commenced on appropriate cardio-protective agents including a statin, appear to go on living with remarkable stability. I accept there are plenty of other changes that are confounders. Nonetheless, at this stage, I believe for patients who are clearly at high risk, as indicated by the diagnosis of coronary artery disease, and for patients demonstrated to have a high- to very high-risk atheroma burden demonstrated on imaging, that statins form an important part of an holistic risk management strategy.

From where I sit, even without any trial data, **for the right patient, they work!**

IMPORTANT POINTS ✓

- Every medication carries risk to the user. It's important to be clear about the benefit *any* medication will have for the patient.

- Although they are among the most studied and prescribed agents in medical history, the use of statins is dogged by controversy and questions. Twenty years of experience tells me that, for the right patients, they work. The question always is: **what are the risks and the benefits for the patient?**

[1]   Scandinavian Simvastatin Survival Study G. Randomised trial of cholesterol lowering in 4444 patients with coronary heart disease: the Scandinavian Simvastatin Survival Study (4S). The Lancet 1994;344:1383-89.

[2]   Rojas-Fernandez C, Hudani Z, Bittner V. Statins and cognitive side-effects: what cardiologists need to know. Cardiology clinics 2015;33:245-56.

[3]   Dobs AS, Schrott H, Davidson MH, et al. Effects of high-dose simvastatin on adrenal and gonadal steroidogenesis in men with hypercholesterolemia. Metabolism 2000;49:1234-8.

[4]   Davidson MH, Stein EA, Dujovne CA, et al. The efficacy and six-week tolerability of simvastatin 80 and 160 mg/day. Am J Cardiol 1997;79:38-42.

[5]   Sathyapalan T, Kilpatrick ES, Coady AM, Atkin SL. The effect of atorvastatin in patients with polycystic ovary syndrome: a randomized double-blind placebo-controlled study. J Clin Endocrinol Metab 2009;94:103-8.

[6]   Swerdlow DI, Preiss D, Kuchenbaecker KB, et al. HMG-coenzyme A reductase inhibition, type 2 diabetes, and bodyweight: evidence from genetic analysis and randomised trials. The Lancet;385:351-61.

[7]   Newman TB, Hulley SB. Carcinogenicity of lipid-lowering drugs. Jama 1996;275:55-60.

[8]   Sultan S, Hynes N. The ugly side of statins. Systemic appraisal of the contemporary un-known unknowns. 2013.

[9]   DuBroff R, de Lorgeril M. Cholesterol confusion and statin controversy. World Journal of Cardiology 2015;7:404-09.

Chapter 8 -
Evaluating and reporting risk

> assessing risk:
  – the significance of calcium
  – features of the atheroma plaque

Today's approach to risk evaluation is, in general terms, related to evaluating factors that have been shown to be associated with increased risk in population studies and then applied to the individual: factors such as age, smoking, presence or absence of diabetes, cholesterol levels. These are the risk factor associations that give rise to **possible** development of a problem based on the observations associated with major adverse coronary events in large population studies.

For the sake of this discussion, I will refer to these risk factors as **'traditional'** risk factors and I will introduce a separate concept, **'plaque-**specific' risk. By this, I mean that there are features which are demonstrated on cardiac CT imaging, particularly relating to the plaque in question. The individual plaque (or plaques) may have a clear and specific impact on the risk of the potential development of a major adverse coronary event but, importantly, the risk is plaque-specific and may not necessarily match up with the risk suggested by the traditional risk factors.

It is important to understand that **both are significant and should be used in combination** in the decision-making related to the best ongoing care and risk modification of an individual patient.

Currently, **there is no standardised, structured approach to the description of risk within cardiac CT imaging.** For previously discussed historical reasons, the emphasis of risk association and imaging of the heart have been principally the domain of calcium scoring, which provides an indicator of the propensity of an individual patient to develop coronary atheroma within the arteries. In this regard, coronary calcification could be considered as a **traditional** risk indicator. This is particularly so with higher range calcium scores. Progressing to CT coronary angiography (the injection of contrast to outline the lumen of the artery, thus providing detail about the structure of individual plaques) gives an opportunity to make an assessment that relates to **plaque**-specific risk.

Regardless of a patient's cholesterol levels, the amount of exercise he or she undertakes (or not), how healthy the person claims his or her diet is, I want to know the health of **that** individual's arteries, not the risk that a population of people with the same characteristics may have. To do this, I believe, we get the most information by using CT to look directly at the arteries.

Coronary calcium score and risk

My practice is to obtain a coronary calcium score. Calcium scoring provides a sensitive indicator to the presence of atheroma. It is an absolute number and there is a significant body of research which supports the premise that the greater the absolute coronary calcium score, then the greater the risk of an event that an individual carries.

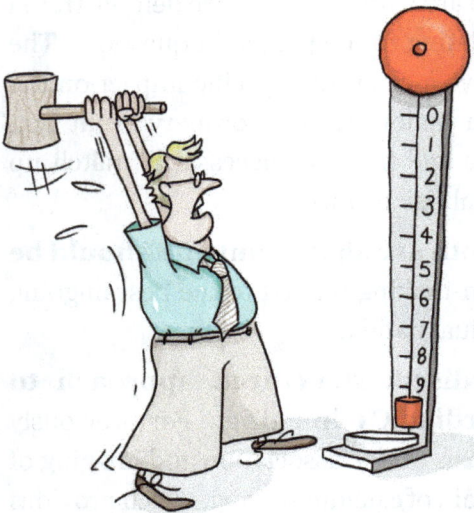

Who knows what calcium score you'll get?

As we have already discussed, **calcium is not the problem** but is an indicator of a potential risk. **The problem is the plaque build-up.** Scavenger cells, the macrophages, try to clean up the cholesterol and, in so doing, can become so 'full' that they burst and spill their contents which include digestive enzymes. The enzymes cause scarring in the artery wall. The build-up of cholesterol, scavenger cells, scar tissue and calcium in the wall of the artery is the plaque. Agatston's early work in demonstrating an association between the amount of calcium present in an individual's arteries and the risk of progressing to a major adverse coronary event means that calcium scoring has become a prominent and sensible marker in risk assessment.

Observational data in relation to people with a zero calcium score is robust. It covers more than 30,000 patients and indicates that a zero calcium score carries a less than one percent chance of a coronary event in a 10 year period[1-3]. This makes **coronary calcium scoring a very powerful negative predictive test** (meaning the condition is not present) in cardiology. Neither a normal stress test (running on a treadmill), nor a normal invasive coronary angiogram (when contrast or dye is injected directly down the arteries) can provide the same assurance, while 'low cholesterol', 'regular exercise', 'good diet', 'watching my weight' and a 'healthy lifestyle' cannot come anywhere near to being as useful in predicting a low risk of an event as does a zero coronary calcium score.

....

This next section is controversial and may cause a negative response from my colleagues who are ardent practitioners of evidence-based medicine and advocates of guidelines. Some of my colleagues, however, will see a line of logic that stitches together patches of evidence where gaps exist.

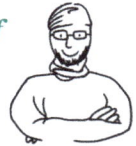

For patients, I hope it provides information that can form the basis of a sensible discussion with their medical practitioners, in order to meet their own particular needs.

....

Calcium as a gatekeeper

Due to this robust body of data, my own practice is to use the coronary calcium score (CCS) in its own right or as a gatekeeper to CT coronary angiography. My feeling is that not everyone needs both a calcium score and a CT coronary angiogram for risk stratification.

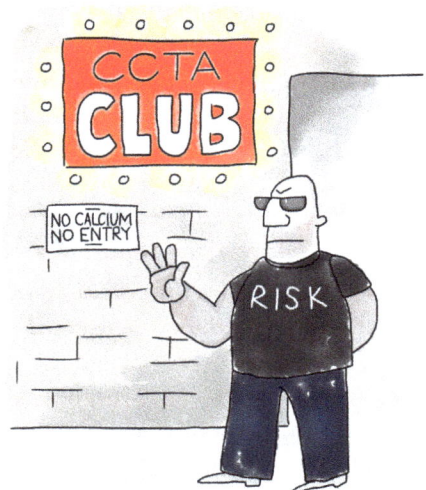

If, however, an abnormality is detected, then it **is** my general recommendation that we progress to CT coronary angiography, to obtain as much information as possible about the health of that patient's coronary arteries.

Current literature and guidelines support the use of CCS alone for risk stratification, particularly for intermediate-risk patients[4].

My own experience, however, is that in certain patients the amount of calcium underestimates the actual plaque burden present. This tends to be the case in younger patients who may have a family history of premature coronary disease, perhaps with elevated triglycerides and non-HDL cholesterol, features of insulin resistance (increased waist to hip ratio) or even a family history of type 2 diabetes. In these cases, the CCS may be low but this may be in the setting of a large non-calcific (cholesterol dominant) plaque burden, such that the patient is likely to carry a much higher risk of a MACE than suggested by the CCS alone.

Until we have clear information from the literature that tells us reliably how to identify those patients, their risk is significantly underestimated by the CCS alone. I'm comfortable with explaining this situation to the patient and allowing the patient to be involved in calcium scoring alone, or calcium scoring followed by CCTA if calcium is present.

Why not CCTA for everyone?

To use a coronary calcium score only has several benefits.

FIRSTLY, in the asymptomatic patient, the literature supports that a zero score is a very reassuring test.

SECONDLY, it provides a lower radiation dose than a cardiac CT (CCS + CCTA) study. At every stage in medicine we need to be asking the question: Is the risk of a particular test outweighed by its benefit? With a low radiation dose from calcium scoring resulting in a zero calcium score, there seems to be little point in subjecting the patient to further radiation when the negative predictive value of a zero calcium score is so low.

THIRDLY, it is a relatively cheap test. Why progress to a more expensive test when the first has already demonstrated a very low risk over the next 10 years?

FOURTHLY, the coronary calcium score requires no contrast, is extremely safe and avoids any potential risk or complication associated with the injection of contrast media or dye.

Importantly, in this setting of asymptomatic patient evaluation, there is no data to suggest that CCTA adds incremental information in risk stratification over and above the CCS. In fact, there is published literature that suggests adding CCTA to CCS adds no benefit[5]. The limitation of that data, however, is that it is observational data from a registry that was not a dedicated study to explore the possible additional benefit of adding CCTA information to CCS information in management and then outcome. Only the degree of stenosis was used rather than including other features of plaque *(discussed later)* that may have added to more precision and a different outcome. Also, there is some data from the same group suggesting that *there is incremental outcome prediction benefit* in adding CCTA to CCS in patients with symptoms[6].

My experience is that if we find calcium on the CCS then, unless we follow up with the CCTA, it is not possible to be clear as to the health of that individual's arteries. *(I discuss this approach in more detail for medical practitioners in Appendix 3)*

There is one other specific practice I have surrounding coronary calcium scoring and that is using fine cut (0.6mm) sections in men who are under 50 years of age and women under 60. Remember, the standard Agatston Score uses three millimetre slices (set by the specifications of the scanner)[7]. So, I'm talking about using thinner slices (available on the modern machines, which were not available to Agatston for his original work) to look at the heart to be more precise in the detection of calcifications.

Coronary calcuim score and coronary event risk (CER)

10 YEAR CER

Baseline coronary calcium score	With diabetes	With metabolic syndrome	With neither diabetes nor metabolic syndrome
0	2.0%	0.8%	0.6%
1-99	8.8%	5.5%	3.5%
100-399	14.5%	12.5%	6.3%
400 or more	16.9%	15.8%	11.3%

Data from average 4-6 year follow-up of patients in the Multi-Ethnic Study of Atherosclerosis (MESA). Dr Malik. Jan 2010.

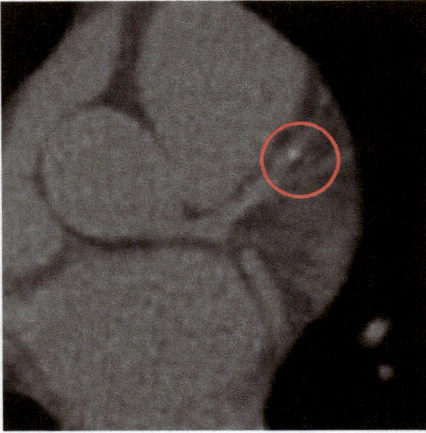

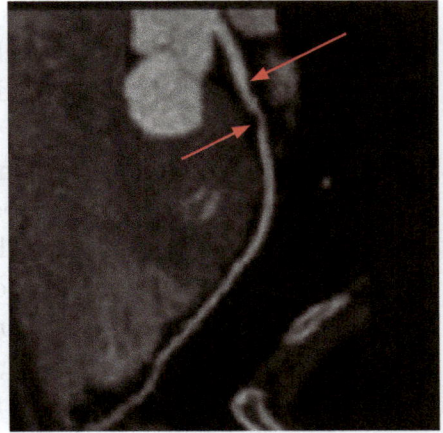

This scan shows a fleck of calcium on the left (a zero score) and the significant cholesterol build-up that was associated with it in a male under 50 years of age.

I use the fine cut because small amounts of calcium may be present that could relate to a build-up of plaque, yet might not be picked up on standard Agatston scoring in which the speck of calcium may not be big enough to register. A zero score in this situation could be erroneous[8]. The likelihood of this misleading zero score becomes less as the patient gets older[9].

Sex and age

As a person ages, that person is more likely to have some evidence of calcium within the arteries. This brings us to the concept of an expected CCS score range for age and sex, or a percentile score for age and sex. It poses the question: *What's an average calcium score for my age and sex?*

Within each age and sex population, there is a distribution. For example, in a group of one hundred 50-year-old-men, the lowest risk 25 men will have a zero calcium score (this is the lowest quarter of scores and called "first quartile"), while the highest risk 25 men will have scores of over 100 (this is called the "fourth quartile"). *(Please refer to the coronary calcium score percentile chart on right[10].)*

By using men at 50 and women at 60 as the cut-off for zero Agatston scores, I am ensuring that a zero calcium score represents the best quartile for that age/sex group and so may not be inadvertently representing a higher risk *(see circles on chart).*

Coronary calcuim score percentile chart

AGE (Years)

	35–39	40–44	45–49	50–54	55–59	60–64	65–70
Men	(479)	(859)	(1066)	(1085)	(853)	(613)	(478)
25th percentile	0	0	0	0	3	14	28
50th percentile	0	0	3	16	41	118	151
75th percentile	2	11	44	101	187	434	569
90th percentile	21	64	176	320	502	804	1178
Women	(288)	(589)	(822)	(903)	(693)	(515)	(485)
25th percentile	0	0	0	0	0	0	0
50th percentile	0	0	0	0	0	4	24
75th percentile	0	0	0	10	33	87	123
90th percentile	4	9	23	66	140	310	362

The number of patients in each group is in parentheses.

It can be seen that a zero calcium score in a younger patient may not necessarily mean that that patient sits in the lowest risk group for age and sex. For example, a zero calcium score for women between 35 and 39 means that, as they age, they could eventually end up in the 25th, 50th or even the 75th percentile for age and sex *(see rectangle on chart)*. In this situation adding in fine slice assessment down to 0.6mm allows improved evaluation by potentially altering where that patient may fit within his/her age-matched cohort. In the setting of a 35–39 year-old woman, some flecks of calcium which do not register as a full score on the Agatston score, would suggest it is possible that patient sits between the 75th and 90th percentile.

An easy example of this is to take a calcium score of 28. On its own this is not a particularly high-risk feature. It carries with it a risk of an event over the next 10 years of approximately 3.5 percent. If, however, we were to obtain a coronary calcium score of 28 in two separate individuals then the significance of that result, when percentiles are taken into account, becomes more obvious.

For a male aged between 65 and 70 years, a coronary calcium score of 28 falls within the first 25 percent for age and sex for that population. This would be considered a relatively low-risk finding and would be unlikely to have significant upward pressure on that risk based on the absolute calcium score alone. *For a female aged between 45 and 49 years,* a coronary calcium score of 28 would fall above the 90th percentile for age and sex. This is a markedly elevated coronary calcium score for age and sex and would have a significant, upward effect on the risk, as assessed by the absolute score alone[1].

So, the absolute coronary calcium score then can be viewed through the prism of the calcium score percentile for age and sex, such that an approximation to a propensity for the development of atheroma can be assessed.

So for primary prevention screening, I generally stop at a zero calcium score for men 50 years or older, and women 60 years or older[2]. For younger patients with significant risk factors, however, I will often progress to a CCTA if there are specks of calcium found on the 'fine cut' (that is 0.6mm slices) even if the Agatston Score (based on three millimetre slices) is zero[3,4].

This discussion has been concerned with traditional risk factors.

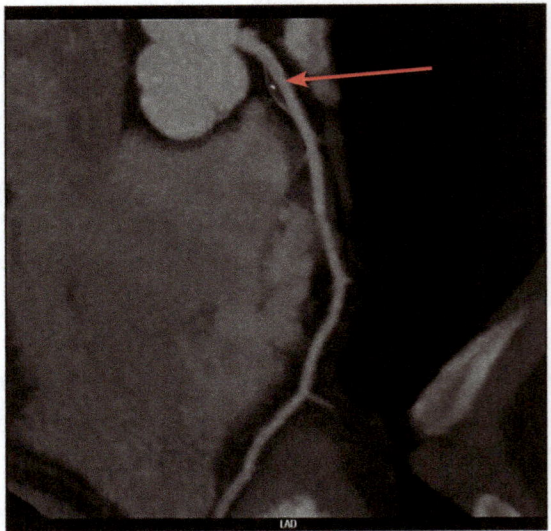

The image for this 30-year-old man with a terrible family history of premature coronary artery disease shows a small speck of calcium at the origin of the LAD (main artery down the front of the heart), although he had a zero calcium score.

This image also shows a large non-calcific plaque with the speck of calcium in the middle of it. For this case obtaining the CCTA shows the real risk for this young man. This is a high-risk plaque and without treatment would lead to this young man following the family tradition!

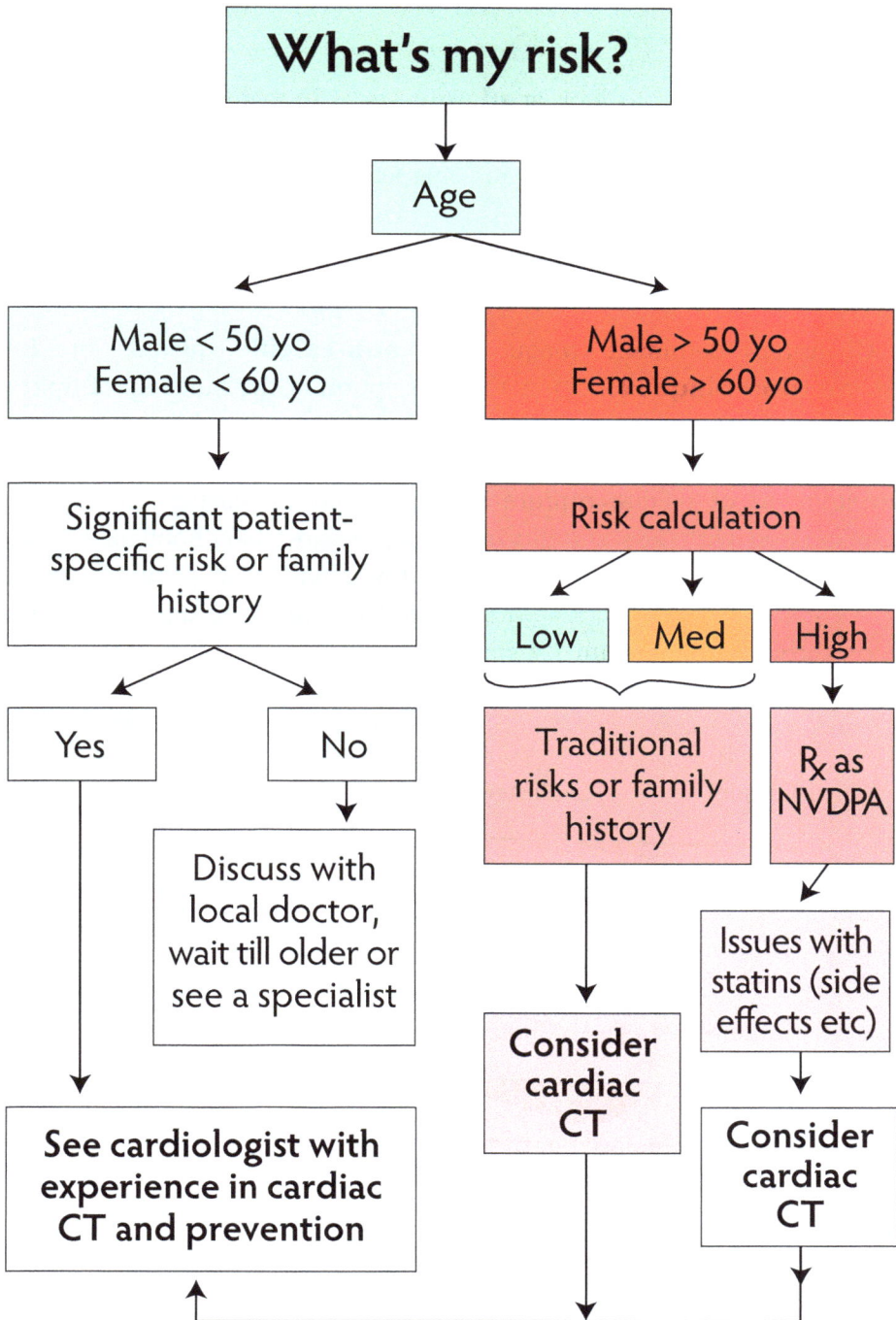

What's my risk?

Age

Male < 50 yo / Female < 60 yo

Significant patient-specific risk or family history

Yes → See cardiologist with experience in cardiac CT and prevention

No → Discuss with local doctor, wait till older or see a specialist

Male > 50 yo / Female > 60 yo

Risk calculation

Low / Med / High

Traditional risks or family history → Consider cardiac CT

R$_x$ as NVDPA → Issues with statins (side effects etc) → Consider cardiac CT

Plaque and risk

The next stage is to look at **plaque-specific** factors. A CCTA, which involves injecting contrast into a vein in the arm, will outline the details of the arteries so that the structure and characteristics of individual plaque can be more thoroughly assessed.

CHOLESTEROL-DOMINANT PLAQUE   The most important issue that I now look for is cholesterol-dominant plaque within the artery.

Cholesterol-dominant plaque, or **non-calcific** plaque or **low attenuation plaque** (LAP), is the description of the build-up of lipid or fat within the plaque. The extent to which this occurs can have a significant bearing on the stability of the plaque. Our understanding around the development of plaque rupture indicates that increasing lipid content is associated with less stability and so a greater likelihood of rupture. Observational study shows that once a low attenuation plaque is greater than eight millimetres in length and two millimetres in diameter (a LAP volume greater than 20mm³), it starts to carry a significant increased risk of event over the next few years.

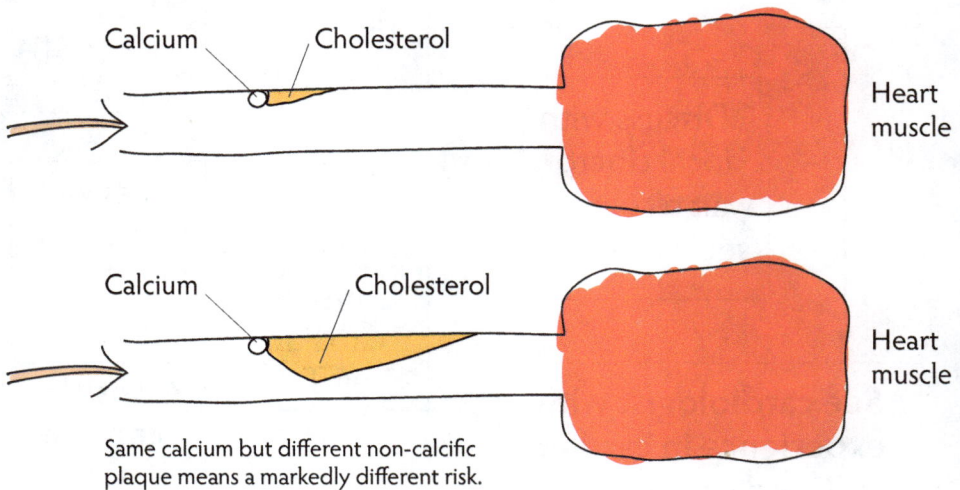

Same calcium but different non-calcific plaque means a markedly different risk.

The diagram shows two spots of calcium in an artery but they point to very different risk profiles due to the amount of associated cholesterol-laden plaque.

This is very important as it is possible to find significant low attenuation plaque in the setting of a low coronary calcium score and relatively low calcium score percentile. In this situation, the risk associated with the individual plaque becomes dominant in the future likelihood of the development of a major adverse coronary event for the individual patient. The significance of this is that, although CCS is well validated for use in risk prediction, it can dramatically underestimate risk in patients who display non-calcific plaque deposition in excess of calcium deposition. This reiterates my point that the most comprehensive assessment of the health of the arteries, if calcium is demonstrated, is the combination of both CCS and CCTA, a complete 'cardiac scan'.

REMODELLING

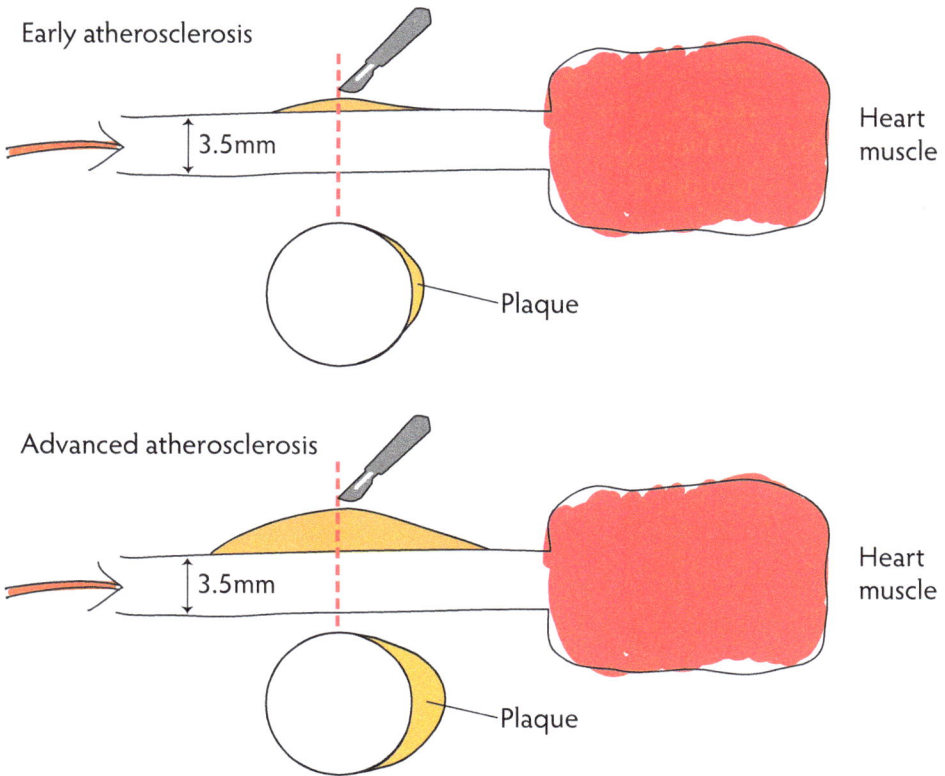

Progression of unfavourable positive remodelling

113

Remodelling is the process in which the vessel changes shape, enlarging to accommodate the build-up of atheroma within the artery wall. Because it can lead to enlargement, it is referred to as **positive** remodelling (although it may not be 'positive' for the patient). Initially there is no encroachment on the lumen (the inside space of the artery), yet it is a process that has been observed to carry with it a significant risk of event. Expansion changes within the artery of greater than 10 percent have been associated with rates of event of 3.5 percent in two years. This is a 15-20 percent risk over 10 years and intermediate- to high-risk of its own.

Significant fatty or low attenuation plaque (greater than 8mm x 2mm), together with unfavourable remodelling, has been observed to be associated with event rates of over 20 percent in two years. This is a 100 percent rate over 10 years and is a very, very high-risk feature.

STENOSIS A further plaque-related feature that warrants assessment in risk evaluation is stenosis or **narrowing.** There is good data suggesting that if there were a narrowing of greater than 50 percent, then the particular plaque involved could have event rates of over five percent per annum. Over 10 years this would be a 50 percent event rate and, of its own, a high- to very high-risk feature.

SITE or LOCATION Lastly, the location of a high-risk plaque is important to factor into a risk assessment. This is common sense but is also backed by data. This supports the premise that the more proximal a ruptured plaque that gives rise to an event is, then the worse the outcome; the more distal and the smaller amount of myocardium at risk, then the better the prognosis.

IMPORTANT POINTS ✓

- Traditional and plaque-specific risk features should be used in combination.
- Coronary calcium scoring is a very powerful negative predictive test.
- Calcium build-up in arteries increases with age.
- Some patients, particularly young ones, may have their risk underestimated by CCS alone. However, thinner slices can pick up calcium in younger patients.
- The CCS percentile for sex and age is useful in risk stratification.
- A high measure of calcium for age and sex increases risk further.
- Features of the plaque that can be considered in relation to increased risk are:
  » the extent to which the plaque is cholesterol-dominant;
  » the extent to which the artery has been remodelled (expanded unfavourably);
  » the extent to which the plaque has caused stenosis (narrowing) within the artery, and
  » the site of plaque.

[1]   Budoff MJ, Shaw LJ, Liu ST, et al. Long-term prognosis associated with coronary calcification: observations from a registry of 25,253 patients. J Am Coll Cardiol 2007;49:1860-70.

[2]   Georgiou D, Budoff MJ, Kaufer E, Kennedy JM, Lu B, Brundage BH. Screening patients with chest pain in the emergency department using electron beam tomography: a follow-up study. J Am Coll Cardiol 2001;38:105-10.

[3]   Budoff MJ, Nasir K, McClelland RL, et al. Coronary calcium predicts events better with absolute calcium scores than age-sex-race/ethnicity percentiles: MESA (Multi-Ethnic Study of Atherosclerosis). J Am Coll Cardiol 2009;53:345-52.

[4]   Latif MA, Budoff MJ. Role of CT angiography for detection of coronary atherosclerosis. Expert Rev Cardiovasc Ther 2014;12:373-82.

[5]   Cho I, Chang H-J, Sung JM, et al. Coronary computed tomographic angiography and risk of all-cause mortality and non-fatal myocardial infarction in subjects without chest pain syndrome from the CONFIRM Registry (COronary CT Angiography EvaluatioN for Clinical Outcomes: an InteRnational Multicenter Registry). Circulation 2012:CIRCULATIONAHA. 111.081380.

[6]   Al-Mallah MH, Qureshi W, Lin FY, et al. Does coronary CT angiography improve risk stratification over coronary calcium scoring in symptomatic patients with suspected coronary artery disease? Results from the prospective multicenter international CONFIRM registry. European Heart Journal-Cardiovascular Imaging 2014;15:267-74.

[7]   Agatston AS, Janowitz WR, Hildner FJ, Zusmer NR, Viamonte JM, Detrano R. Quantification of coronary artery calcium using ultrafast computed tomography. J Am Coll Cardiol 1990;15:827-32.

[8]   Aslam A, Khokhar US, Chaudhry A, et al. Assessment of isotropic calcium using 0.5-mm reconstructions from 320-row CT data sets identifies more patients with non- zero Agatston score and more subclinical atherosclerosis than standard 3.0-mm coronary artery calcium scan and CT angiography. Journal of cardiovascular computed tomography 2014;8:58-66.

[9]   Raggi P, Gongora MC, Gopal A, Callister TQ, Budoff M, Shaw LJ. Coronary artery calcium to predict all-cause mortality in elderly men and women. J Am Coll Cardiol 2008;52:17-23.

[10]   Raggi P, Cooil B, Callister TQ. Use of electron beam tomography data to develop models for prediction of hard coronary events. Am Heart J;141:375-82.

[11]   Budoff MJ, Hokanson JE, Nasir K, et al. Progression of coronary artery calcium predicts all-cause mortality. JACC: Cardiovascular Imaging 2010;3:1229-36.

In the next chapter we look at bringing precision to the reporting of an individual's risk stratification.

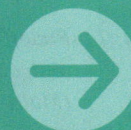

Chapter 9 -
Reporting a clear message

IN THIS CHAPTER WE LOOK AT 👁

> the importance of the report

Currently, there are two major data sets relating to cardiac CT. The first outlines coronary calcium scoring and strongly supports the use of calcium as a marker for cardiovascular risk. The second set relates to the reliability of CT coronary angiography for an **anatomical** or structural description of the coronary arteries.

The Society of Cardiac Computed Tomography, in the latter part of 2014, released its guidelines for interpretation and reporting CCTA[1]. This document focussed predominantly on the interpretation of CT coronary angiography and on the description around a detailed reproducible format of reporting for the findings anatomically. Although calcium scoring is mentioned, there is no comment regarding risk interpretation in the reporting guidelines.

In my practice, I review a patient who, if indicated, is then prepared for a cardiac CT with appropriate heart-rate-regulating medication. I review that patient's scan so that I have a feel for the state of the arteries. This means that when I consult with the patient after the scan, I have the benefit of seeing, if you like, the picture of that person's heart.

I believe a picture 'is worth a thousand words'. **The opportunity to make a risk assessment, having looked at the health of someone's arteries, is an extraordinary opportunity and, to my way of thinking, is without question, beneficial.** This is because it is very hard to report the anatomical findings within an artery and expect the referring doctor, who may not necessarily have expertise in cardiac CT imaging, to understand what the anatomical description means in regard to risk.

Let me clarify this with an example. A report may read:

"calcific and non-calcific plaque and changes consistent with early remodelling demonstrated in the proximal left anterior descending with no evidence of flow limitation".

This anatomical description could be absolutely correct. However, unless the doctor who will be acting on that report understands exactly what this anatomical description means, the doctor will not be able to put it into an appropriate context for risk modification for that patient. If the doctor reads *"no evidence of flow limitation"* and mistakenly considers this reassuring, then he or she would be wrong and the patient may be under-treated for future cardiovascular risk.

The unit I work within reports according to the guidelines of the SCCT. It has been my observation, however, that we do not report in a way that necessarily allows a specialist without expertise in cardiac CT imaging, or a general practitioner who has referred a patient for risk stratification, to have an appropriate grasp of the risk that the patient may actually carry, based on the scan features alone.

Following are some excerpts from reports that have been generated from our unit and sent back to the referring doctor; I have been a co-reporter. I offer them to show that, for a medical practitioner not fully aware of all the subtleties related to risk within calcium scoring and CT coronary angiography, these reports do not provide clear guidance for risk management in the individual patient. Below each report I have added a comment to aid your understanding.

REPORT: *Heavy calcification over proximal coronary arteries, precluding further assessment with CT coronary angiography. Agatston score 1649.5*

COMMENT: This is a very high coronary calcium score and would suggest high- to very high-risk of a MACE.

REPORT: *Moderate plaque burden. Areas of mild to moderate stenosis in the LAD. A severe stenosis in the LAD could not be excluded. Functional/ clinical correlation suggested if clinically indicated.*

COMMENT: It is hard to tell what sort of risk this patient carries. Is it mild to moderate? It is almost certainly increased but it's not easy to know for someone unfamiliar with the terminology and technology. The features would suggest high- to very high-risk of a MACE.

REPORT: *Eccentric mixed plaque in the distal left main / proximal LAD causing <50% luminal narrowing. There is no other visible disease. Although the actual volume of disease is small, placing the patient between the 25-50th percentiles for age and gender, the location of disease is concerning. Aggressive risk management is recommended.*

COMMENT: This is the beginnings of a risk comment, although risk is not actually mentioned. Suggesting aggressive risk management probably means it looks pretty high risk on the scan but what is 'aggressive risk management'? Is it statin therapy to target? What if statin is not tolerated? Does the patient need to lose weight? Exercise? Is it to treat diabetes or pre-diabetes? Is dialysis/plasmaporesis required to remove cholesterol from the blood stream? Is it a stent? Is it cardiac surgery? Is it enrolment in a trial for one of the new lipid-lowering agents? Does it include family screening?

The point is that the report of a scan, often generated by a reporting specialist(s) who may not have seen or spoken to the patient, cannot of its own dictate how a patient is managed. Surely, it is better to give the referring clinician a clearer indication of the risk that may be suggested by the scan, and then let the practitioner decide what management is required, based on a comprehensive understanding of the patient's clinical details.

From this background, with a realisation that cardiac CT imaging (combining CCS and CCTA) offers an insight into the health of the arteries and so potentially provides information that could improve risk management for that individual patient into the future, I realised that reports that gave risk guidance to the referring doctor could be beneficial for patient care.

As I have mentioned earlier, the language that we use around cardiovascular risk in medicine is low, intermediate and high risk of a major adverse coronary event. Low risk is up to 10 percent risk of an event in 10 years; high risk is greater than a 20 percent risk of an event in 10 years, and intermediate risk is in between.

From a practical perspective, I believe that if we can produce reports from cardiac CT imaging which use this sort of language, then the information will be accessible and relatable to the referring doctor, regardless of whether or not that practitioner has expertise in cardiac CT imaging. This would then benefit the patient.

The C-PLUSS Model for risk evaluation

Using the features that I look for *(as outlined in the previous chapter)*, I use a simple acronym that allows me to be more precise in reporting risk evaluation:

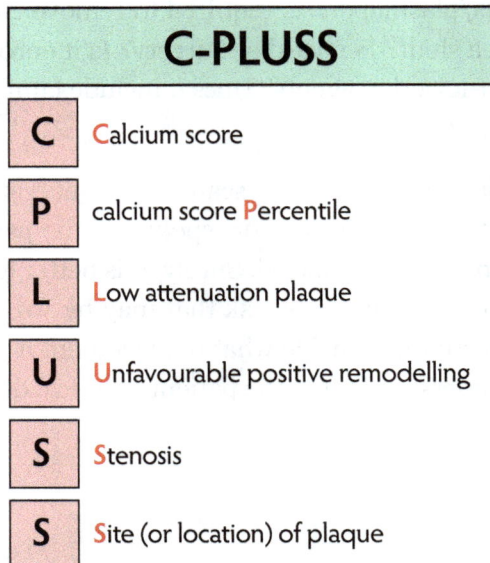

C-PLUSS	
C	Calcium score
P	calcium score Percentile
L	Low attenuation plaque
U	Unfavourable positive remodelling
S	Stenosis
S	Site (or location) of plaque

I report cardiac CT in terms of anatomy using the standard convention and in keeping with the SCCT guidelines. I add the C-PLUSS comment when speaking with patients and also in my explanation back to the general practitioner who will be caring for the patient into the future. In the following example, you will see that the features are described as "been observed to be associated with". This is a deliberate use of language, as the basis of the C-PLUSS model is derived from observational studies.

Standard Report

The CCS is 550 distributed over the left main (32), the LAD (294), the RCA (156) and Cx (68). There is proximal and mid-LAD mixed plaque demonstrating positive remodelling with stenosis up to 50%. There is proximal Cx mixed plaque, less than 20%. There is proximal RCA mixed plaque, with positive remodelling less than 50% stenosis and mixed plaque at the origin of the PDA less than 20%.

Three vessel disease without flow limitation.

Risk Comment

The CCS is high (550). This has been observed to be linked to risk of a MACE of 10 to 15% in 10 years. The CCS percentile is >75. This would suggest an increase in risk based on CCS alone by severalfold, and carry an increased lifetime risk.

Presence of significant non-calcific plaque burden, with associated unfavourable positive remodelling, has been observed to be associated with event rates up to 20% in 2 years. This is a very high-risk feature.

The location of disease in the Left Main, proximal LAD, Cx and RCA is concerning due to the territory potentially affected by an event.

The features of this cardiac CT study have been observed to be associated with high to very high (>>20% risk in 10 y) CV risk. This information should be combined with an evaluation of the patient's other CV risk factors for a comprehensive risk profile to help in guiding further management.

The report deliberately avoids vague terms such as "aggressive treatment" and describes risk features that are present at the time of scanning, without comment on other traditional risk factors. It is up to the referring doctor to take the cardiac scan information and apply it to the patient as appropriate.

To the average reader, all this may seem hard work and too complicated to worry about. The reason I include it, however, is for you. If you do choose to undertake cardiac CT scanning to evaluate your own risk, particularly if you have invested your own money to do so, I think you will want to make sure the report you receive is what you paid for and something from which you will actually benefit. So, feel free to ask your doctor and/or the provider of the scan if a structured risk comment is being used in the reports. If not, you know where to direct them. I have included in the appendix a copy of a paper I co-authored on this topic in Cardiology Today. It provides more detail and supporting references.

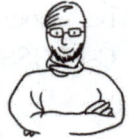

IMPORTANT POINTS

- Describing what is there is the anatomy.
- Interpreting the anatomy is the risk.
- Understanding the patient is clinical.
- Combining the anatomy with risk and the clinical picture gives management.

[1]   Leipsic J, Abbara S, Achenbach S, et al. SCCT guidelines for the interpretation and reporting of coronary CT angiography: A report of the Society of Cardiovascular Computed Tomography Guidelines Committee. Journal of cardiovascular computed tomography; 8:342-58.

In the next chapter we discuss bringing a practical approach to a patient's risk stratification.

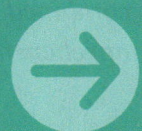

Chapter 10 -
Holistic risk evaluation

IN THIS CHAPTER WE LOOK AT

> bringing together the traditional and plaque-specific risks in a practical approach

I have tried to make clear the distinction between population-based or traditional associations with the development of coronary artery disease in an individual and the plaque-specific issues. Most importantly, the evidence base that we doctors work from in terms of risk management is firmly based on population-type assessments. As discussed previously, Framingham is the most recognisable example of this type of risk evaluation. There are, of course, other risk calculators available. For example, there is an Australian website *(http://www.cvdcheck.org.au/)* which allows an individual to plug in his/her own parameters to arrive at a population-based risk calculation.

I have also tried to demonstrate that, by scanning the heart, we can make an assessment of a person's cardiovascular risk based on the individual propensity to deposit cholesterol within the arteries. And, I have alluded to the importance of focal cholesterol deposition in the arteries, such that one centimetre of plaque in the entire coronary tree may be the defining feature for an individual's life.

So far, I have tried to demonstrate that imaging is a **valuable addition** in assessing an individual's cardiovascular risk that may be calculated from population-based associations alone. This is what I do in my own practice. Importantly, because there is substantial data supporting Framingham-style risk calculation, we have to combine it as part of the basis of our formulation of a risk calculation in an individual. The approach needs to be holistic. Just because a patient may have low-risk atheroma burden, it doesn't mean we can ignore elevated blood sugar levels or high blood pressure.

My proposition, however, is that we can then take that information and add to it the specific findings from cardiac CT imaging so that we can bring precision to an individual patient's risk stratification, moving from a population-based probability of an event to a far more specific evaluation of the health of an individual patient's arteries.

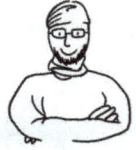

In my opinion, the ability to combine the Framingham-type risk (traditional) of an individual patient with the imaging of his or her arteries (plaque-specific) allows the most comprehensive risk evaluation for an individual, not only for the present but also for possible future cardiac problems. Cardiac CT imaging will lead to a conclusion that the features observed on the scan could be low-risk features, intermediate-risk features, high-risk features or very high-risk features. This needs to then be married to the Framingham-type risk calculation. An approach to this follows.

LOW-risk plaque features matched to traditional features

LOW – LOW In the setting of a patient with low plaque risk cardiac CT features, who also has a low traditional risk factor profile based on Framingham, there is really nothing to do. This patient is at very low risk of a cardiovascular event in the next 10 years.

LOW – INTERMEDIATE If low plaque risk features are suggested from the cardiac CT scan in the setting of an intermediate traditional risk factor profile on Framingham, then such things as lifestyle modification, regular blood testing and regular lipid profiling may be appropriate, with consideration of repeat scanning in the future.

LOW – HIGH High-risk traditional factors need to be managed as per National Vascular Disease Prevention Alliance (NVDPA) guidelines. Some individual patients may have reservations about medication without more detail or perhaps have experienced side-effects from previous medication. For those patients, if the cardiac CT scan demonstrates low-risk plaque features in the setting of a high traditional risk factor profile based on Framingham, then this presents an interesting situation in which the individual appears to have no localised substrate or promoters for plaque formation but nonetheless would sit within a population that carries a high risk. In the short term, the finding of clear arteries probably implies a low risk which is likely to be more robust the older the patient. In this situation, interpretation by the referring doctor, in association with a thorough evaluation of the patient's risk profile, is critical.

I would discuss these findings in significant detail with the patient. If the risk factor profile is significant enough, we would start lifestyle modification and therapy regardless or, in some situations, we might agree to rescan the heart at a short time interval (say two years) monitoring for any changes in atheroma burden. This is an evidence-free zone, so an understanding of the processes and the application of some common sense, with the engagement of the patient in the process, I believe, is the best way forward.

INTERMEDIATE-risk plaque features matched to traditional features

INTERMEDIATE – LOW In the setting of intermediate-risk plaque features demonstrated on cardiac CT imaging but a low traditional risk factor profile as suggested by Framingham modelling, there are two ways forward and engaging the patient in the discussion is critical. This is also an evidence-free zone and, as such, I believe, best handled with as much information as possible and the involvement of the patient in the decision-making.

Some patients would ideally wish to avoid medication, predominantly for philosophical reasons. Some patients would want to avoid statins, for example, due to side-effects. In an intermediate-risk plaque features cardiac CT scan with a low-risk factor profile, if a patient did want to avoid medication, then significant attention to lifestyle modification and consideration of repeat scanning in three to five years could be a reasonable option. Repeat coronary calcium scoring will give an appreciation of progression of CCS which has been linked to outcome. A rate of increase of CCS of greater than

10 to 15 percent per annum carries a significantly higher risk of an event compared with less than these percentages[1,2].

Other patients may see the opportunity to minimise their risk by taking a tablet as the best way forward. In Australia, there are Pharmaceutical Benefits Scheme guidelines which dictate a medical practitioner's ability to prescribe statins that are supported financially by the government. Conversation, therefore, has to be held in the context of the patient's ability to access a subsidy. Those who do not meet the criteria will need to be aware that they will bear the statin cost.

....

"For how long do I take statins, Doc?"

When I recommend to the patient that he or she will benefit from taking statins and aspirin, the patient will often ask "For how long?" I say, "For life". This has a deliberate double meaning, of course.

Unfortunately, our current therapy really only works while the patient is taking the medication. A course of tablets might be a possibility for the future but it is not current reality. This means that the medication will need to be taken for the remainder of the patient's life. However, the aim is not for people to live forever; the objective is for people not to die prematurely, especially while they still have a contribution to make or there are things they want to see or do. I tell my patients that when they are bed-bound in a nursing home, being fed soft food and having someone help them go to the toilet, they can spit out the tablets and let nature take its course!

....

INTERMEDIATE – INTERMEDIATE For a patient with this profile, the same conversation as just described needs to be held.

INTERMEDIATE – HIGH If intermediate-risk plaque features are found in the setting of a high-risk factor profile as suggested by Framingham-type evaluation, then this patient needs to be treated as per the NVDPA guidelines.

Intermediate risk is not that reassuring for the patient. Imagine if you were told that you had a 15 percent chance of being in a plane crash in the next 10 years. It is incomprehensible! Yet, we accept an intermediate risk of major adverse coronary event. That assumes no change in patient risk factors, such as gaining weight, decreasing exercise, blood sugars creeping up or, one that we can't control, increasing age!

....

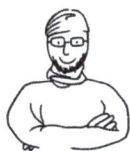

Remember, if we were to take 100 people with intermediate patient risk (15 percent risk of an event in 10 years), then 15 of those 100 people are actually at high risk and 85 are at low- to intermediate-risk. If a cardiac scan finds one of the 15, by demonstrating features that have been observed to be associated with a high- to very high-risk, then my feeling is that the person needs to be treated based on the health of his/her arteries, not the calculated risk. This situation is a reminder that we don't fully understand the process of the build-up of cholesterol in the arteries and that there is inaccuracy in dealing with an individual based on population-fit alone.

....

HIGH-risk plaque features matched to traditional features

HIGH – LOW or INTERMEDIATE If high-risk plaque features are demonstrated on cardiac CT imaging in the setting of a low- to intermediate-traditional risk factor profile, then I treat these patients as high-risk and apply the NVDPA guidelines. This is a situation when what's happening in the arteries cannot be predicted by looking at the patient and is available only from looking at the arteries themselves.

HIGH – HIGH If high-risk plaque features are demonstrated on cardiac CT imaging in the setting of a high-risk traditional factor profile, as suggested by a Framingham calculation, there is no question that this person needs to be managed as per the NVDPA guidelines. The cardiac CT imaging in this situation confirms the necessity for appropriate risk factor modification with specific effort to treat cholesterol levels to accepted targets.

If cardiac CT imaging demonstrates **very high-risk features,** particularly a stenosis of greater than 50 percent, then regardless of the risk factor profile, this patient should be seen by a cardiologist with experience in cardiac CT and interest in prevention, for further assessment and possible testing.

- **Low-risk cardiac CT features** in the setting of:
  - » **Low-risk Framingham** factor profile – nothing to do.
  - » **Intermediate**-risk factor profile – modify lifestyle, consider repeat scanning in five to 10 years.
  - » **High**-risk factor profile – manage as per guidelines. If that is not possible, may repeat scan in two years, or start treatment but may accept lower targets with fewer side-effects.

- **Intermediate-risk cardiac CT features** in the setting of:
  - » **Low-risk Framingham** factor profile – modify lifestyle and may consider repeat scanning in three to five years, or start treatment but may accept lower targets with fewer side-effects.
  - » **Intermediate**-risk factor profile – manage as per guidelines.
  - » **High**-risk factor profile – manage as per guidelines.

- **High-risk cardiac CT features** in the setting of:
  - » **Low- or intermediate-risk Framingham** factor profile – suggest treating as high risk.
  - » **High**-risk factor profile – manage as per guidelines.
  - » **Very high**-risk factor profile – suggest cardiologist review; remember family screening may be appropriate.

let's be clear about risk

Stuck in the middle

From a practical perspective, the two extremes of low risk and high or very high risk are the easiest to deal with. Low risk requires little more than reassurance, a plan for ongoing lifestyle care and consideration of the role of future reassessment. Similarly, high- or very high-risk features dictate that therapy should be undertaken.

The grey area lies in intermediate risk. This is where an understanding is needed, not only of the limitation of the data that is available to guide us, but also of the factors that may be associated with the risk, whether they be population-based, traditional associations which can be modified or plaque-specific factors within the arteries of the individual. Either way, I believe this intermediate-risk situation allows for thoughtful discussion and decision-making around the best way forward, with the opportunity to involve the patient in that process.

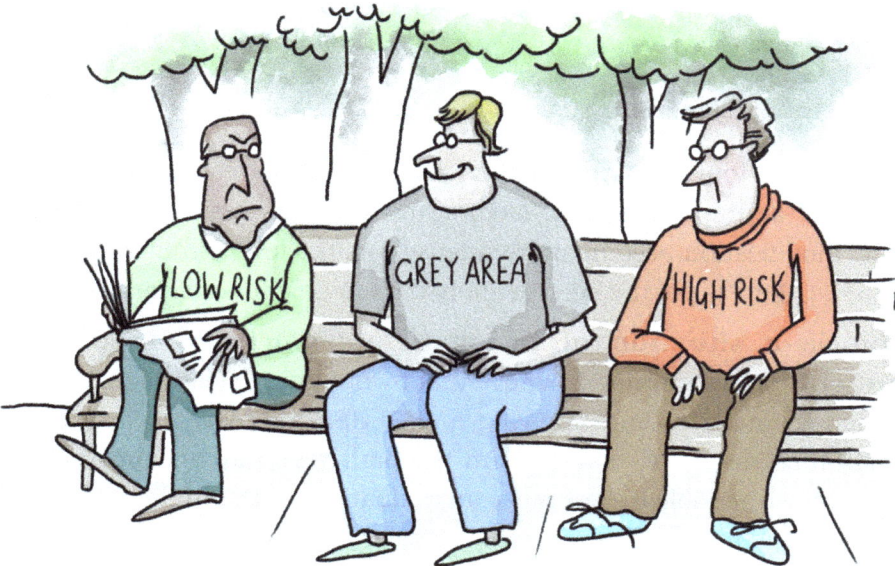

It is my experience that to have imaging available to indicate the health of someone's arteries is extremely valuable, as it takes the discussion away from a population-based probability to a specific atheroma burden within an individual, the latter being far more significant in terms of patient involvement and acceptance.

Clear indicator

By the end of a Framingham-type risk assessment, combined with a cardiac CT and C-PLUSS risk assessment, there is a very clear indication as to whether there is presence or absence of atheroma burden. If there is a build-up of cholesterol in the arteries, we can be specific and clear as to whether the build-up is mild, moderate, severe or very severe. With that information, we can then be very precise about our objectives in management and continuously measure and adjust our intervention to match the extent of the process and the underlying risk.

How much more sense does this make compared with just taking a cholesterol tablet because one's cholesterol is a bit elevated? Wouldn't you rather your doctor manages the observable processes occurring in your body than treats a test result?

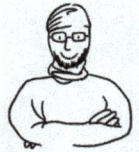

As the level of our risk assessment increases, efforts to reach targets, accept side-effects, address other risk factors and more aggressively undertake lifestyle modification become more intense. As the level of our risk profile diminishes, there is not the need to apply the same rigour or intensity.

This is a situation of trying to appropriately match the treatment to the needs. I believe that by obtaining a cardiac CT image of someone's arteries and applying a C-PLUSS approach to appreciate the risk, then matching that up with the patient's Framingham-type risk calculation, we are able to best make an evaluation for that individual's care at that time and into the future.

IMPORTANT POINTS

- The more information the better for making a decision.
- Low risk is straightforward to manage.
- High risk is straightforward to manage.
- Intermediate risk requires discussion and thought to determine the most appropriate care.
- The most holistic care comes from combining **traditional population** generalisation with **individual visualisation!**

[1]   Callister TQ, Raggi P, Cooil B, Lippolis NJ, Russo DJ. Effect of HMG-CoA reductase inhibitors on coronary artery disease as assessed by electron-beam computed tomography. N Engl J Med 1998;339:1972-8.

[2]   Raggi P, Callister TQ, Shaw LJ. Progression of coronary artery calcium and risk of first myocardial infarction in patients receiving cholesterol-lowering therapy. Arterioscler Thromb Vasc Biol 2004;24:1272-7.

The two particular situations in the context of very high-risk findings which are discussed in the next chapter will be of particular interest to readers who enjoy detail, as well as to medical practitioners.

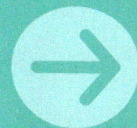

Testimonial

I have had moderately high cholesterol levels for the past 30 years and have them checked annually by my GP. Given this history, I recently sought advice from my GP regarding a test that I could have to identify any early signs of heart disease. My GP recommended Dr Warrick Bishop as he specialises in the early detection and prevention of heart disease, which is exactly what I was seeking.

Based on my history and lifestyle, Dr Bishop indicated that my risk of heart disease would be at the lower end of the scale but, to provide further peace of mind for the next 5 to 10 years, I could have a cardiac CT scan. Dr Bishop clearly explained the minimal risks associated with the procedure and in layman's terms described how the CT scan takes a series of individual x-rays that are combined to make a 3D picture of the heart and arteries, thereby identifying any build-up of plaque on the artery walls. Dr Bishop advised me upfront that this procedure was not covered by Medicare. However, the moderate cost was far outweighed by the peace of mind that it provided.

The CT scan was very simple and took only a few minutes plus a total of 30 minutes monitoring before and after. My appointment started at 9am and I was back at work before 10am. The worst part of the procedure was not having my usual cup of coffee first thing in the morning!

I would gladly recommend Dr Bishop to my family and friends and I would not hesitate to have a cardiac CT scan in the future.

Conrad Lennon

Chapter 11 -
Particular high-risk findings

> two ends of a spectrum:

- patients with very high calcium scores for their age

- patients with relatively low calcium scores but risky cholesterol build-up

Before moving away from these considerations of high risk, I would like to discuss two situations in the context of very high risk findings and the manner with which I deal with them:

1. a **very high coronary calcium score** or a very high calcium score percentile falling above the 90th percentile for age and sex, and

2. when there are **very high-risk plaque features combined with a low coronary calcium score.** This is when there is a large cholesterol-laden (non-calcific) plaque while the coronary calcium score would suggest a low risk.

Both require special attention.

1. High coronary calcium score

In the setting of a very high coronary calcium score, or one greater than the 90th percentile for age or sex, I view these patients as sitting well outside the normal range and therefore, they require more than our standard lipid profile for assessment. Let's face it: if an individual is clearly outside the normal range, why would you test that patient using tests for the average population?

Our current testing for lipids covers total cholesterol, triglycerides, high density lipoprotein, low density lipoprotein, non-high density lipoprotein and total cholesterol to HDL ratio. The term 'lipoprotein' refers to the carrier of the cholesterol in the blood stream. Left to its own devices, cholesterol in the blood stream would behave like cream in milk; it would clump and float to the top. So, to be able to move cholesterol around the body through the blood, it needs to be attached to a protein that can carry it and keep it under some control.

The proteins that carry the cholesterol are known as *lipo* (meaning fat) proteins. They have different structures and different roles. Some move cholesterol into the tissues; some take cholesterol away from the tissues and to the liver. This means that not just the total amount of cholesterol is important, but also the type of protein that is carrying it is significant. The standard panel of blood tests checks for three carriers of lipid within the bloodstream when research tells us that 15 to 20 different carriers exist. If we are checking for only three out of 15-20 carriers of cholesterol, what impact do the other lipoproteins have? My practice in this higher risk group is to obtain a broader evaluation of the lipid panel. The tests I obtain include the lipid panel for what would be considered standard practice for the average patient as well as novel (extra) markers.

Standard tests:

TOTAL CHOLESTEROL (TC) This is a measurement of all cholesterol in the blood stream, regardless of the lipoprotein that is carrying it around. It doesn't differentiate between 'good' and 'bad' cholesterol but it is the number that patients seem best able to remember.

TRIGLYCERIDES (TG) This is a marker of 'free fats' and is best measured in the fasting state, otherwise it can be quite significantly affected. Often triglycerides will be elevated in people who have a predisposition to put weight on around the belly. They will also be raised in patients who are pre-diabetic or type 2 diabetic.

HIGH DENSITY LIPOPROTEIN (HDL) This is generally considered a protective form of cholesterol which has a role in slowing (even reversing) deposits of cholesterol into the arteries. As such, the higher the HDL level, generally, the more favourable the outlook for the individual.

TOTAL CHOLESTEROL TO HDL RATIO (TC:HDL) This is a way to take the absolute cholesterol measurement and put it in the context of how much 'good cholesterol' is present. Observational studies suggest that there is a balance between deposits of cholesterol into the arteries and removal of cholesterol from the arteries. A ratio can be an effective way of trying to understand that balance. A high total cholesterol, for example, matched with a high HDL level could yield a low ratio and, therefore, may not be particularly atherogenic, or tending to promote the formation of fatty deposits in the arteries. Conversely, a fairly average total cholesterol level could be matched with a particularly low HDL level, yielding a high TC:HDL ratio which is considered more concerning.

NON-HIGH DENSITY LIPOPROTEIN (non-HDL) This is a grab-bag measurement of everything that is not HDL. Without having to separate all the lipid-carrying proteins into subtypes, it gives a general appreciation of cholesterol being carried through the blood stream of the person. In general terms, the higher the non-HDL number, the more atherogenic it is believed the profile will be.

LOW DENSITY LIPOPROTEIN (LDL) This is considered the 'bad cholesterol' and is certainly the one about which the vast majority of research has been undertaken and where the targets of our therapy lie.

For the high-risk patient, I also order:

APO-LIPOPROTEIN B (ApoB) This is a measurable lipoprotein fragment that gives us an idea of the size of the LDL particle. There has been clear demonstration of LDL existing in more than one form. It can exist in a 'large fluffy' form which seems to be less atherogenic than a 'small dense' form which seems to be more closely related to the development of atheroma.

The higher the ApoB level, the more 'small dense' particles and the higher the risk of an event[1,2].

LIPOPROTEIN (a) (LPa) This is another carrier of lipid through the blood stream and, in fact, it is a component of LDL cholesterol. Lipoprotein (a) has only recently started to attract more attention, as it has not been investigated as extensively as other particles. However, it is observed to be linked to premature coronary artery disease and certainly has been demonstrated as an association for the development of coronary artery disease[3].

I also check some other factors outside the lipid measurements:

HOMOCYSTEINE This is a product of an enzyme system used in energy generation. Research suggests that elevated levels of homocysteine can be linked with increased rates of plaque formation[4].

THYROID FUNCTION Plenty of data support the proposition that an under-functioning thyroid gland is linked with changes in the lipid profile, particularly elevated triglyceride levels[5]. Making sure that the thyroid is functioning properly is common sense in this setting.

VITAMIN D Sets of data support that vitamin D deficiency, particularly over a prolonged time, can have a negative effect on the lipid profile and can be linked with increased cardiovascular risk[6]. This is easy to remedy, so knowing if there is a deficiency is worthwhile.

FASTING BLOOD SUGAR This is an important indicator in assessing whether or not the patient is diabetic, or on the path towards diabetes[7].

FASTING INSULIN This is a test rarely undertaken but I find it extremely valuable, particularly in combination with the fasting blood sugar level test. Insulin is the hormone that the body produces to deal with carbohydrate metabolism and so controls sugar levels. It is also produced when the body has had a good feed and wants to store that energy (food, as fat) for later.

HOMA[8] This is a calculation from the fasting insulin and fasting blood sugar levels to give an indication of the *insulin resistance* of an individual. This is important as some people are more insulin-resistant than others. This means that, for a given exposure to carbohydrate, they will require more insulin to control the blood sugar level. The more insulin-resistant the individual, the higher the insulin levels, the higher the triglycerides and the greater the chance of progressing to diabetes in the long term.

2. Low calcium – high-risk plaque features

The second specific situation is the high-risk plaque dominated by cholesterol (non-calcific) in the setting of a patient with a low overall coronary calcium score. This refers to a plaque containing a small amount of calcium (which would give a low calcium score) but that has a big lump of soft cholesterol build-up associated with it. This is a plaque that could be associated with a high risk in the future, a risk far greater than estimated from the calcium score alone.

There is very little data around this. However, there is observational work that points toward low attenuation plaque dominance being associated with elevated non-HDL cholesterol levels[9].

I often see this in families and specifically in families who appear to have a predisposition to premature coronary artery disease and/or diabetes. In these patients, I have found a high incidence of non-HDL cholesterol, which is in keeping with previous observations, but I have also found that there is an elevated fasting insulin and there are features of insulin resistance, as demonstrated by an elevated HOMA. I have seen this in 5 to 10 percent of patients in whom I have observed these phenomena. These are unpublished data but certainly interesting.

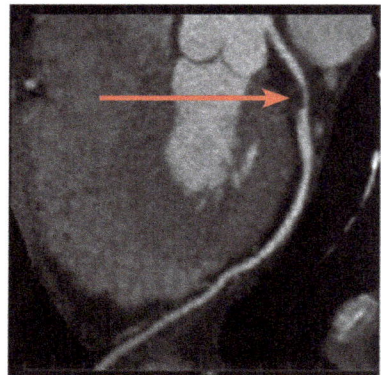

Low calcium, cholesterol dominant high-risk plaque. The arrow points to cholesterol-rich plaque in the major artery down the front of the heart. There was barely a speck of associated calcium.

IMPORTANT POINTS ✓

- There appears to be a spectrum of plaque formation characteristics:
  - » at one end there is a propensity to calcification (lots of calcium), and
  - » at the other end, non-calcific plaque is dominant (not much calcium).
- Extra testing may be warranted in both of these situations.

[1] St-Pierre AC, Cantin B, Dagenais GR, et al. Low-density lipoprotein subfractions and the long-term risk of ischemic heart disease in men: 13-year follow-up data from the Quebec Cardiovascular Study. Arterioscler Thromb Vasc Biol 2005;25:553-9.

[2] Yusuf S, Hawken S, Ounpuu S, et al. Effect of potentially modifiable risk factors associated with myocardial infarction in 52 countries (the INTERHEART study): case-control study. Lancet 2004;364:937-52.

[3] Ference BA, Yoo W, Alesh I, et al. Effect of long-term exposure to lower low-density lipoprotein cholesterol beginning early in life on the risk of coronary heart disease: a Mendelian randomization analysis. J Am Coll Cardiol 2012;60:2631-39.

[4] Robertson J, Iemolo F, Stabler SP, Allen RH, Spence JD. Vitamin B12, homocysteine and carotid plaque in the era of folic acid fortification of enriched cereal grain products. CMAJ 2005;172:1569-73.

[5] Rizos CV, Elisaf MS, Liberopoulos EN. Effects of thyroid dysfunction on lipid profile. Open Cardiovasc Med J 2011;5:76-84.

[6] Jorde R, Grimnes G. Vitamin D and lipids: do we really need more studies? Circulation 2012;126:252-4.

[7] Association AD. Diagnosis and classification of diabetes mellitus. Diabetes Care 2014;37:S81-S90.

[8] Matthews D, Hosker J, Rudenski A, Naylor B, Treacher D, Turner R. Homeostasis model assessment: insulin resistance and β-cell function from fasting plasma glucose and insulin concentrations in man. Diabetologia 1985;28:412-19.

[9] Nakazato R, Gransar H, Berman DS, et al. Relationship of low- and high-density lipoproteins to coronary artery plaque composition by CT angiography. J Cardiovasc Comput Tomogr 2013;7:83-90.

How to find high-risk patients in a crowd is discussed in the next chapter.

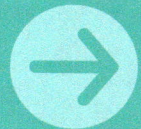

Testimonial

Dr Warrick Bishop and the CT angiogram investigation have become immensely important in my treatment of patients with potential cardiac disease. As a practising GP, a simple test like this with a high level of accuracy is a great tool for treating disease and encouraging lifestyle change. This book is a good read for anyone. It can save a life. What an amazing thing that is.

John Saul GP, Lauderdale, near Hobart

Chapter 12 -
Being ahead of the game

IN THIS CHAPTER WE LOOK AT 👁

> finding the high-risk patients in a crowd

As discussed earlier, the approach to coronary artery disease historically has been driven by responding to symptoms late in the process, or has been guided by risk calculators that have limitations to their application.

I believe we can define high-risk patients before they have an event.

From a pragmatic point of view, the objective is to be ahead of the game so that we know who has a significant atheroma burden and who is at significant risk, before an event. My objective in trying to reduce risk for individual patients is to prevent them from having an out-of-hospital cardiac arrest that leads to death or to substantial damage to the heart muscle, outcomes that are irreversible, costly and, I believe, potentially avoidable. We are not necessarily attempting to avoid stenting or coronary artery bypass grafting. These technologies work very well when required. What we want is more control, with the aim of avoiding the unexpected out-of-hospital heart attack trauma; **we want to stabilise the plaque to prevent rupture.**

If we screen and identify potential high-risk individuals and if we institute cholesterol-lowering therapy and therapy to thin the blood[1], then instead of having a catastrophic myocardial infarction, the patient may be likely to present with a more stable picture, such as chest pain on exertion or shortness of breath. Having been educated as part of the process of being identified as a high-risk patient, the person knows to present immediately, which has its own positive prognostic benefit[2,3]. If by starting lipid-lowering therapy and aspirin therapy in the high-risk group, we are able to alter the way coronary artery disease presents, then I believe we have an opportunity to **significantly reduce the rates of acute myocardial infarction and so lessen the emotional and financial burden** to individuals and to the community.

At the time of writing, there exist American and European guidelines and an Australian position statement for use of CCS in risk stratification, although there are no guidelines for using cardiac CT (CCS and CCTA) for screening. Here are some general pointers I use.

Structured screening

I look to screen men who are 50 years of age unless there is a significant history of premature coronary artery disease or significant traditional risk factors that may suggest this person is at marked increased cardiovascular risk compared with the standard population of 50-year-old men. In the latter group, the potentially increased risk patients, I would then recommend screening 5 to 10 years earlier than the age that the youngest family member was affected by coronary artery disease. I believe these patients, who are potentially high risk, would benefit from review by a cardiologist with an interest and expertise in the area. In these situations, particularly with the significant family risk patients, I take considerable time weighing up pros and cons of screening together with family history and an appraisal of their traditional risk factors. There is an individual complexity to this which cannot be covered by the scope of this book.

Premature coronary artery disease:

I always ask if there is a history of coronary artery disease in the family and I'm particularly interested in knowing if there is a male in the family younger than about 50-55 years old or a woman younger than about 60 who has had a coronary event. If there are family members who have had heart problems but are much older, then it is not premature nor will it have a significant effect on the risk of the rest of the family. Smoking will bring forward the likelihood of an event; the rule of thumb I use is by about 10 years. So a 62-year-old woman who is a heavy smoker and has a cardiac event is only borderline for premature coronary artery disease. However, a non-smoking, male younger than 50 years old who has an event is without question a candidate for premature coronary artery disease.

Screening for disease is not a new concept. We regularly have our blood pressure checked; women are used to pap smears and mammograms, and men are used to screening for prostate issues. Screening for bowel cancer using detection of invisible amounts of blood in the stool (occult blood) and, if indicated, endoscopy, have become widespread. Screening for **risk** of coronary artery disease is undertaken regularly already, by general practitioners using Framingham-style risk calculators. As discussed earlier, there are limitations to probability-based screening for disease. There is a clear distinction between finding cancer cells through a biopsy and trying to predict the likelihood of a problem from related factors. This is the difference between screening **for** the disease and screening for the **risk** of the disease.

Currently, there is no structured screening approach for the detection of coronary artery atheroma, although coronary heart disease is the single largest killer in Australia and responsible for some of the most significant health costs in the country.

Let's recall our risk terminology: Less than 10 percent risk of an event in 10 years is considered low risk; greater than 20 percent risk of an event in 10 years is considered high risk, and in between is considered intermediate risk. On average, most men move into the intermediate-risk category about the age of 50. This means that if we were to follow one hundred 50-year-old men for 10 years, 15 of them would have an event and 85 would not. Again, as discussed previously, current practice is not to treat routinely at intermediate-risk, as the treatment of the 85 people who would not benefit dilutes the statistical significance for the 15 people who would benefit. We have considered this acceptable in medicine. Yet, if you or I were among 100 people standing in an airport lounge and we were advised by the captain that we were at intermediate-risk of having a plane crash in the next 10 years, that is, a 15 percent chance that our plane might crash, **wouldn't we find this completely unacceptable?**

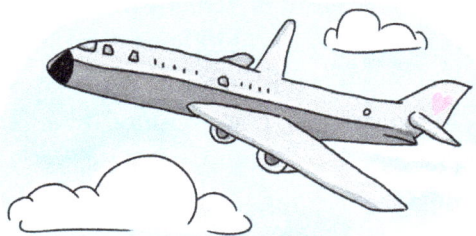

The crux of the issue then becomes: **Can we take those one hundred 50-year-old men at intermediate risk**, with 85 who are unlikely to have a problem in 10 years and the 15 who are likely to have a problem in 10 years, **and be more precise about our management of them by using cardiac CT imaging?** I believe we can.

Recommendation

Let me remind you of the calcium score percentiles discussed earlier. It turns out that at 50 years of age, 25 percent of men will have a zero calcium score; the 50th percentile score is 16 (this is the score right in the middle of the range) and the 75th percentile score is 100 (this is the score marking three-quarters of the way to the highest score). Based on absolute scores, we could quite reasonably make a cut-off: scores above 100 for 50-year-old men are high enough and risky enough that we should consider treatment. Remember, in Chapter 8, I explained how I believe the extra information obtained by looking at atheroma and plaque characteristics can be very valuable and help provide a more complete picture.

So if we use coronary calcium scoring only on those 100 men to start with, we should identify 25 with a zero score. This is based on the percentile information available and also discussed in Chapter 8. These men, based on all data available, are likely to have a very low risk of an event over the next 10 years and require nothing further in terms of cardiovascular risk assessment, assuming their other risk factors remain stable.

For the remaining 75 patients then, we have undertaken a calcium score and will go on to coronary angiography to yield a 'full' cardiac CT. The results of this 'full' cardiac CT will demonstrate that 15 people have high- to very high-risk features, **the 15 percent.** These are the 15 people out of the 100 with whom we would start appropriate treatment. Most, but not all these individuals, will have calcium scores that fall between the 85th and 100th percentile and, if we wanted to include the 75th to 85th percentile to be safe, then there are 25 patients (75th percentile and above) whom we would consider treating. Treating above the 75th percentile is supported to some degree by the literature, which suggests a five year event rate of 10 percent (or a 20 percent 10 year risk) that means that only 25 patients need to be treated to avoid one event[4]. This makes it a reasonable clinical and economic cut-off. As discussed, and based on my own observations, there are some patients for whom a full cardiac CT will show a far higher risk than indicated by their calcium score alone. It seems to represent a relatively small percentage, so let us say for the sake of this calculation that it is five percent of patients. We can only find these patients by progressing to CT coronary angiography, the injection of the dye.

Is it worth the risk? We always have to be mindful of weighing the risk-to-benefit of any testing for an individual. The risks here are from radiation exposure as well as anaphylaxis from the injection of contrast. The risk of allergic reaction causing death is 1 in 100,000. As an aside, your risk of dying in a motor vehicle accident or by gunshot in the United States is in the order of 1 in 10,000!

Our cardiac CT risks are acceptable when dealing with obtaining as much information as possible in patients who may have a minimum of 20 per cent risk of a MACE in 10 years.

Ultimately, this is the decision for the individual patient to make with his/her doctor. My own experience is that having the most information gives the best platform from which to make choices for the patient's heart health future.

And yes, if you are wondering, I have had a cardiac CT. For me, the knowledge was worth the risk.

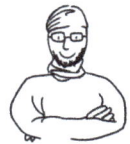

So now we have:-

- used calcium scoring and/or coronary angiography on 100 patients;

- yielded 25 with a zero score – no further action;

- undertaken 75 full cardiac CTs and defined:

  » the 15 with the highest calcium scores who are likely to have a heart attack in the next 10 years;

  » 10 who sit between the 75th and 85th percentile who run an increased risk of heart attack particularly over the next 15 years;

  » 5 to 10 who have features on their cardiac scan which are

substantially higher risk than suggested by their calcium score alone (a subset who could have a MACE contrary to their calcium score alone), and

» about 45 with 'in-between' findings.

This all seems to make sense, so why isn't it being done on a regular basis?

Big picture

An issue that has prevented this approach is that cardiological services are running to maximum capacity and are busy dealing with the complications of coronary artery disease to such an extent that there is little opportunity to step back and look at the big picture.

In the local public hospital in the city where I live, I have offered to be part of the cardiac CT reporting service and also have offered to establish a premature coronary artery disease intervention clinic. At such a clinic, I suggested, I would review patients who had had events early in their lives and,

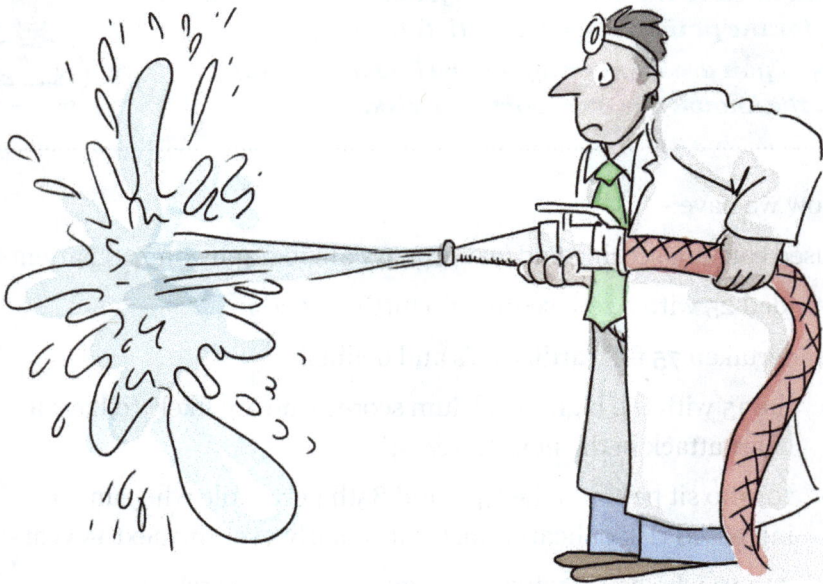

from there, try to screen their relatives in the hope of finding high-risk patients who could benefit from early intervention. I would also look to review patients with increased specific risks, particularly very raised cholesterol levels as seen in familial hypercholesterolaemia. I have been advised that those particular services are not required but assistance on the acute angioplasty roster (the roster for dealing with out-of-hours heart attacks) would be helpful. This situation is probably replicated across this country and across other countries.

The irony is that local health services are so busy putting out fires, they do not have the capacity to stop to see if they can prevent the fires from starting in the first place.

Stress tests

Stress testing is not considered standard practice for screening populations[5]. It is acceptable to check your blood pressure, your cholesterol and other risk factors but there is no standard recommendation for the general population to undergo stress testing. My observation is that occasionally some patients will come for stress testing in the context of risk stratification. I believe this provides some reassurance but it is not necessarily good medicine. (Re-read the introduction if you need a reminder of the potential shortfall of stress testing for telling us the health of the arteries.)

It is interesting to note, however, that there are certain circumstances when stress testing is regularly undertaken: insurance companies still request stress testing; the Confederation of Australian Motor Sport (CAMS), the governing body for motor racing, requires stress testing; the Antarctic Division requires stress testing for people heading south; some offshore workers need to fulfil criteria by their occupational health and safety divisions which include stress testing and, most interestingly of all, the Civil Aviation Authority in Australia (and possibly other parts of the world) still rely on stress testing for evaluating risk of commercial and private airline pilots.

Stress testing will only pick up evidence of narrowed coronary arteries – very late in the process. And then, based on its sensitivity (the percentage of affected subjects that are actually detected by the test), it only picks up the problem at a rate of 75-80 percent, meaning that it will miss one-in-five to one-in-six occurrences[6].

Cardiac CT sensitivity, however, is over 98 percent. This means it might miss only one in 50, making it a very sensitive test[7].

As well as not being particularly accurate, the stress test makes no appraisal of non-flow-limiting coronary atheroma burden which has been demonstrated to be the culprit for coronary occlusion (by rupture of the plaque leading to blockage from the formation of a clot in the artery) in more than 40 percent of cases.

This means, if stress testing detects 75 percent of narrowed arteries accurately and zero percent of non-narrowed arteries, and if 60 percent of heart attacks occur on narrowed arteries, stress testing is detecting 75 percent of 60 percent of the plaque that will lead to a problem, giving a pick-up rate of less than 45 percent (60 percent x 75 percent). A toss of a coin provides a better detection rate (50 percent) by chance alone!

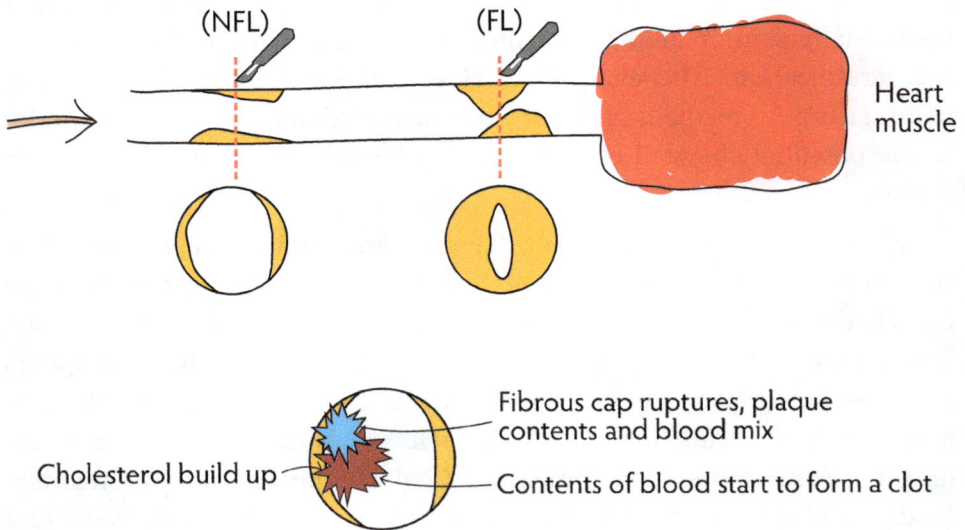

(NFL)   (FL)   Heart muscle

Cholesterol build up — Fibrous cap ruptures, plaque contents and blood mix

Contents of blood start to form a clot

A reminder of non-flow-limiting and flow-limiting plaque and plaque rupture in the artery.

The resulting lack of data means that institutions, such as those already mentioned, are undertaking screening processes which I believe are inadequate. From my own personal safety perspective, I would much rather know that the pilot of the next plane in which I fly has had a cardiac CT scan and has been appropriately assessed, not that he has been able to run for six to nine minutes on a treadmill without any symptoms, a year ago.

To give you an example of this:

I have a patient, Bill F, who, in the context of a family history of premature coronary artery disease, requested cardiac CT imaging at the age of 48. Scanning demonstrated a high coronary calcium score, in fact, above the 90th percentile for age and sex. The CCTA suggested possible narrowing of the circumflex artery. As an aside, we scanned other members of his family and we are appropriately risk- managing them, although their risk was not as high as Bill's.

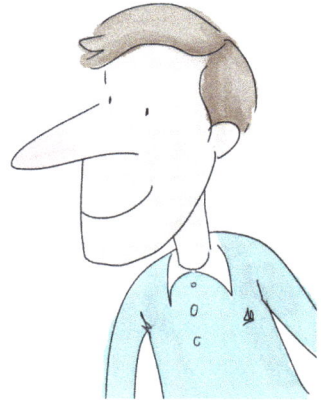

Bill, after also undergoing screening bloods for high-risk factors, ended up taking aspirin, statin, nicotinic acid, ACE inhibitor, vitamin D and fish oil. He undertakes regular exercise and keeps an eye on a reduced carbohydrate eating guideline. Unfortunately, Bill did not tolerate statin well. Still, we have persisted with as much statin as he can tolerate, a very low dose every second or third day.

In the context of not being able to treat as we had hoped, nor achieve the desired lower lipid levels, we discussed repeat coronary calcium scoring as an indicator of whether or not we had been able to slow the progress of his underlying atheroma deposition. We undertook repeat coronary calcium scoring about four or five years after the initial scan. This demonstrated a compounding rate of change per annum of greater than approximately 25 percent, suggesting that we had not been able to control the progression of his atheroma burden as we would have liked. Ideally, it should have been at a rate of change of less than 10-15 percent per annum[8]. We agreed that there was some sense in undertaking stress testing as a potential indicator of progression that could lead to narrowing. *Please note, this is different to using stress testing to define risk. In this situation we already knew the risk from the cardiac scan and used the stress testing to assess if any of the arteries had narrowed over time.*

The electrocardiogram (ECG) demonstrated some change suggestive of narrowed arteries but there was no evidence of regional wall motion abnormality demonstrated on echocardiography (that is, the heart muscle worked well, suggesting good blood supply to the majority of the heart). We repeated the test about a year later with similar results, with no lessening in exercise capacity.

Another year on, we repeated the stress echocardiogram. On this occasion, it clearly demonstrated the presence of regional wall motion abnormality (the muscle 'cramps' from lack of blood and literally becomes stiff, failing to move properly) affecting the posterior wall, most likely affected by the circumflex artery. Bill, because of his excellent exercise capacity, had some mild shortness of breath but performed very well on the test. Nonetheless, the extent of affected muscle was such that I believed we should progress to invasive coronary angiography for consideration of potential revascularisation.

Within the week, Bill had undergone invasive coronary angiography and had a stent inserted into the proximal circumflex artery which resulted in a full re-establishment of blood flow to that area of myocardium. He was back at work several days later. There was no damage to his heart. He resumed full work and full exercise capacity, and is again wrestling with trying to take statins. We plan to continue with follow-up stress testing.

Bill represents, I believe, one of the potential 15 out of the 100 who would have otherwise been "in the crowd" of intermediate risk had we not identified him. His alternative scenario may have been sudden cardiac death or to have presented with a heart attack which could have led to a terrifying ride in the back of an ambulance, Accident and Emergency time, out-of-hours call for the invasive angiography unit to be opened, to be followed by an expensive ICU stay. Damage to his myocardium might have prevented him from returning to the exercise he enjoys, limited his lifestyle, kept him from work and, if the damage were significant, may have required implantation of a defibrillating device. The costs – both emotional and financial – could have been enormous.

IMPORTANT POINTS

- If we take one hundred 50-year-old men, we know about 15 will have a MACE in the next 10 years.

- If we cardiac CT scan the 100, we can find the 15 with the unhealthy looking arteries and treat them appropriately, potentially cutting the heavy emotional and financial costs significantly. We can also find the ones who are at low risk, regardless of their cholesterol level or family history.

- To some degree these are largely unchartered waters. However, my clinical experience is that having as much information as possible for an individual allows us to navigate between the islands of evidence-based medicine.

- Remember, stress testing is not a screening test for high risk atheroma burden. It is a screening test for narrowed arteries that limit the flow of blood, causing ischaemia (lack of blood flow) and therefore will only pick up some problems late in the process, sometimes too late.

[1]   Chow BJW, Small G, Yam Y, et al. Prognostic and Therapeutic Implications of Statin and Aspirin Therapy in Individuals With Nonobstructive Coronary Artery Disease: Results From the CONFIRM (Coronary CT Angiography Evaluation For Clinical Outcomes: An International Multicenter Registry) Registry. Arterioscler Thromb Vasc Biol 2015.

[2]   Tummala SR, Farshid A. Patients' Understanding of their Heart Attack and the Impact of Exposure to a Media Campaign on Pre-Hospital Time. Heart, Lung and Circulation 2015;24:4-10.

[3]   Austin D, Yan AT, Spratt JC, et al. Patient characteristics associated with self-presentation, treatment delay and survival following primary percutaneous coronary intervention. European Heart Journal: Acute Cardiovascular Care 2014;3:214-22.

[4]   Blaha MJ, Budoff MJ, DeFilippis AP, et al. Associations between C-reactive protein, coronary artery calcium, and cardiovascular events: implications for the JUPITER population from MESA, a population-based cohort study. The Lancet;378:684-92.

[5]   Greenland P, Gaziano JM. Clinical practice. Selecting asymptomatic patients for coronary computed tomography or electrocardiographic exercise testing. N Engl J Med 2003;349:465-73.

[6]   Banerjee A, Newman DR, Van den Bruel A, Heneghan C. Diagnostic accuracy of exercise stress testing for coronary artery disease: a systematic review and meta-analysis of prospective studies. Int J Clin Pract 2012;66:477-92.

[7]   Hoffmann U, Bamberg F. Is Computed Tomography Coronary Angiography the Most Accurate and Effective Noninvasive Imaging Tool to Evaluate Patients With Acute Chest Pain in the Emergency Department?: CT Coronary Angiography Is the Most Accurate and Effective Noninvasive Imaging Tool for Evaluating Patients Presenting With Chest Pain to the Emergency Department. Circulation: Cardiovascular Imaging 2009;2:251-63.

[8]   Raggi P, Callister TQ, Shaw LJ. Progression of coronary artery calcium and risk of first myocardial infarction in patients receiving cholesterol-lowering therapy. Arterioscler Thromb Vasc Biol 2004;24:1272-7.

In the next chapter we discuss the unwelcome visitor, chest pain. Before moving on to that, let's ask the question: "What makes a good screening test?"

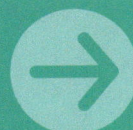

what makes a good screening test?

The role of CT imaging as a screening test is discussed often in the book. An understanding of some aspects of testing will make it easier to understand why I feel CT is such a great test and why I am comfortable recommending it to my patients.

When we consider any test for a patient, there are criteria we use to assess that test:

We want to know:

- how **sensitive** it is – how good is it at **finding** what we are looking for, and

- how **specific** it is – if we find something, will it be **what** we are looking for?

This is possibly best understood as an example. Let's imagine you want to screen for gold nuggets (atheroma) in your back yard. Your screening tool (your test) is a metal detector (CT scanner). There are 100 pieces of gold in your back yard.

If you use your metal detector and find 95 of those pieces, then your tool (test) has found 95 out of the 100 and is about 95 percent sensitive. Alternatively, if you use your metal detector and find 10 of those pieces then your tool (test) has found 10 out of the 100 and is around 10 percent sensitive.

In medical terms, 95 percent sensitivity would be a very good test to find the condition under evaluation; a 10 percent sensitivity is not a good test.

Now, while scanning with the metal detector you may find other metal objects, such as old bottle lids or tin cans or nails. Let's assume there are 1000 of these other metal objects in your back yard. Let's say your detector picks these up at a rate of 95 percent. Now you have found 950 pieces of metal including the 95 pieces of gold. So your specificity (are you finding what you are specifically looking for?) is 95 pieces of gold out of 950 pieces of metal found, which is 95/950 x 100 as a percent and equals 10 percent.

In medical terms, 10 percent specificity is not considered very good as we would want to avoid results that can mislead us.

If by altering the settings on the metal detector, we can reduce the detection of metal other than gold, then we might detect 100 objects of which 95 are gold. We now have a specificity of 95 percent and this is very good.

It is often the case that as sensitivity goes up, specificity goes down.

So, what makes a good screening test?

The following is based on a paper by C. Herman MD (2006)[8], with the points from the Herman paper in bold:

The disease in question should:

- **constitute a significant public health problem, meaning that it is a common condition with significant morbidity and mortality.** There is no question that coronary artery disease ticks this box.

- **have a readily available treatment with a potential for cure that increases with early detection.** Again, coronary artery disease ticks this box; we have medications, balloons and stents as well as surgery.

The test for the disease must:

- **be capable of detecting a high proportion of disease in its pre-clinical state.** Cardiac CT has a sensitivity of over 95 percent. In fact, cardiac CT specificity is also over 95 percent.

- **be safe to administer.** I use the coronary calcium score as a gatekeeper. This is a very safe test, does not use contrast and requires low radiation. Only if this is not normal would I then suggest injecting contrast (severe adverse reaction in 1:100,000 which is still very low risk and achievable with a low radiation exposure).

- **be reasonable in cost.** Using the gatekeeper approach, a CCS is inexpensive ($300 or less) and will be valid for at least 10 years. This is cheaper than yearly cholesterol measurements with medical appointments over the same time, for example. Progressing to CCTA to obtain more information, for say $1000 in total, will allow very specific decisions to be made for the individual over at least the next 10 years. One hundred dollars per year to provide the most appropriate care seems good value to me.

- **lead to demonstrated improved health outcomes.** A substantial portion of this book covers the importance of evidence in medicine and the situations that can arise limiting the available evidence. In this situation, I believe the question should be considered specific to the patient: *Can we demonstrate an improved management strategy for the individual in question?* My experience is that there is no doubt that a clear appreciation of the health of the arteries allows the most appropriate care for the individual. High risk, low risk, need for statins or not, and other questions can be resolved, leading to improved decision making for the patient.

- **be widely available, as must the interventions that follow a positive result.** Recent years have seen improvements in technology such that cardiac CT is now broadly available in major centres and those same centres would have cardiological services to deal with adverse findings.

....

My feeling is that cardiac CT ticks all the boxes. However, it is up to patients and their doctors to discuss the patient-specific issues.

....

[1]   Herman C. *What Makes a Screening Exam good? Virtual Mentor* 2006;8:34-37.

[2]   American Medical Association Council on Scientific Affairs. *Commercialized Medical Screening (Report A-03).* Available at: *http://www.amaassn.org/ama/pub/category/13628.html.*

Chapter 13 -
Investigating chest pain

IN THIS CHAPTER WE LOOK AT 👁

> investigating chest pain and shortness of breath:
- recent onset, unstable angina
- longer onset, stable angina

One of the most commonly recognised signs of a heart problem is chest pain. This unwelcome visitor can come in many guises and can result from a variety of causes, with the most life-threatening being associated with the heart or the lungs. The pain itself has many variations from a severe stab to crushing, burning or a dull ache.

Essentially there are two ways people will present with chest pain. The first scenario is when the chest pain 'hits' very suddenly and the person is taken to an Accident and Emergency Department (A&E). This is described as a possible **unstable angina.** In the second, which is less acute and less sudden, patients will often describe a symptom on exertion such as shortness of breath or chest pain, symptoms that may suggest possible **stable angina.** Most commonly this presentation is seen through the consulting rooms of a cardiologist.

Sudden onset

Having arrived at A&E, the patient will be evaluated, an IV access (a plastic needle in the vein that allows direct injection into the blood stream) in an arm will be established, bloods taken, oxygen and aspirin given (often with a 'spray under the tongue') and an ECG ('dots' are attached to the chest to measure the electric signal of the heart) will be acquired.

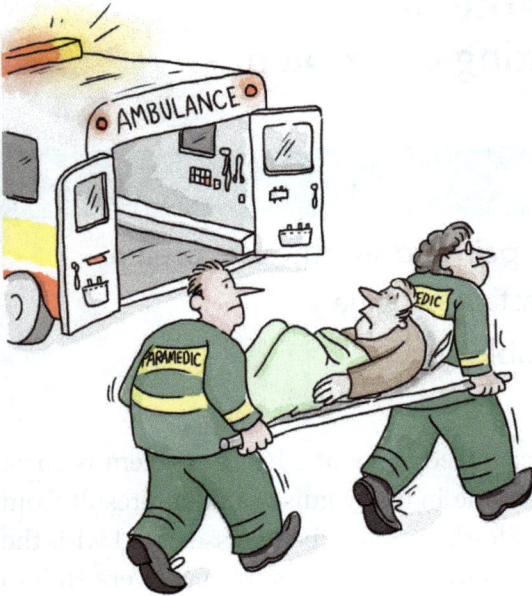

If there is clear evidence that the patient is having a heart attack, then the patient needs immediate intervention and in most large centres will be taken for an invasive coronary angiogram, followed by the implanting of a stent to re-establish blood flow. If that is not available, then there may be protocols in place to administer special drugs which essentially break down the clot within the artery and re-establish flow. *There is no question that this is an effective and appropriate treatment.*

If the patient is not having a heart attack, then the A&E process is to determine whether or not the situation is high-risk heart-related. Serial ECGs and serial blood tests are taken. Changes on an ECG may show ischemia, or shortage of blood flow to the heart. Subtle changes at the time of the first ECG may show dynamic change with the second or third ECG, thus building a case that there is the possibility of a shortage of blood flowing to the myocardium. These ECGs become very important in risk stratification. Concerning changes in the first ECG or dynamic changes certainly suggest the patient is at high risk and there is no question that the person should be admitted to hospital for further evaluation. This situation is called **unstable angina** or an **acute coronary syndrome.**

If the ECG is not changing, significance moves to the blood tests. One of the blood tests which is specifically used in our era is called a **troponin.** A troponin level is an indicator of a particular protein that is released by the heart when it is under stress. Generally, if there are dynamic ECG changes, then the troponin will most likely be elevated. Troponin becomes more useful when there are no ECG changes and the history is not necessarily typical. Research shows that troponin is a good negative predictor; a negative troponin suggests the patient has a low risk of event in the next 30 days[1].

It is this group of patients, with normal ECG and negative troponin chest pain presenting to A&E, that I would like to discuss in more detail.

In hospital

These patients are not necessarily showing high-risk features at the time of presentation but nonetheless may have coronary artery disease as the cause of their pain. They can be a significant burden to an A&E department and it is not infrequent that these patients are admitted to medical or cardiology units for further assessment. When this happens, there are inherent costs that will impact in the longer term on the medical service of that area. Certainly, the time spent in A&E for these patients waiting for a bed can mean that the patient contributes to bed block in the A&E; bed block issues are becoming more problematic across the country in both public and private centres. There is, of course, an associated cost with remaining in A&E until admission and then, at the time of admission, there is a cost per day of being in hospital, potentially in a monitored location on a cardiology ward.

Generally, the plan is to have these patients investigated as soon as possible. However, by virtue of the unpredictable nature of the onset of chest pain, some patients will present on Friday nights, Saturdays or Sundays when standard testing is not routinely undertaken. Some of those patients will remain in a hospital bed for several days waiting for further evaluation prior to discharge, subsequently increasing the cost of their stay.

Usual tests

There are several different ways of testing the patient. Often it will hinge on the availability of a particular service.

It is easy and simple to undertake **exercise stress testing**. This is when a patient runs on a treadmill and an ECG is acquired during that exercise. Changes in the ECG trace are used to indicate a problem. This is a relatively cheap test. It is reassuring for the medical staff in relation to the discharge of the patient.

Stress testing using echocardiography (using ultra sound to take pictures of the heart), looking at how the heart muscle contracts with exercise in association with the ECG, is also relatively simple. It is more costly than the standard exercise testing because it requires echocardiography as part of the test. However, it is more precise and more reliable.

The other test that is sometimes used is **nuclear medicine scanning.** This uses a radioactively labelled marker to give an indication of where blood is flowing in the heart. Often this requires a visit over two separate days for the patient to be assessed as to whether or not the flow to the heart is normal. This test is more expensive in Australia than the previously mentioned two tests, with similar sensitivity and specificity to stress echocardiography.

Increasing attention is being given to the role of **CCTA imaging** in this setting and a number of trials have suggested its safety and utility[2-4].

Lastly, in some situations, the person, having arrived at A&E, will be admitted to hospital and will then undergo **invasive coronary angiography.** Often it is the availability of particular resources that will determine whether or not a patient progresses to this. It may also depend on the person's ability to exercise, or it may rest with the inclination of the clinician looking after the patient. Invasive coronary angiography, however, is the most expensive of the mentioned tests and is not without risk. One in 1000 to 1:2000 cases can be complicated by a serious event.

In practice: cardiac imaging

Having outlined these scenarios, I would like to offer my thoughts on where CCTA imaging may be beneficial in dealing with people presenting to A&E with chest pain.

As noted above, studies have shown that this modality is safe. While it seems that there is not a great deal of cost saving in using cardiac CT imaging, there may be a statistically significant reduction in time spent in hospital. The recent studies which have looked at this in most detail include the Romicat[5] and Philadelphia studies[6]. Although these are both important studies, they do not lend strong weight to changing our current approach[2,3].

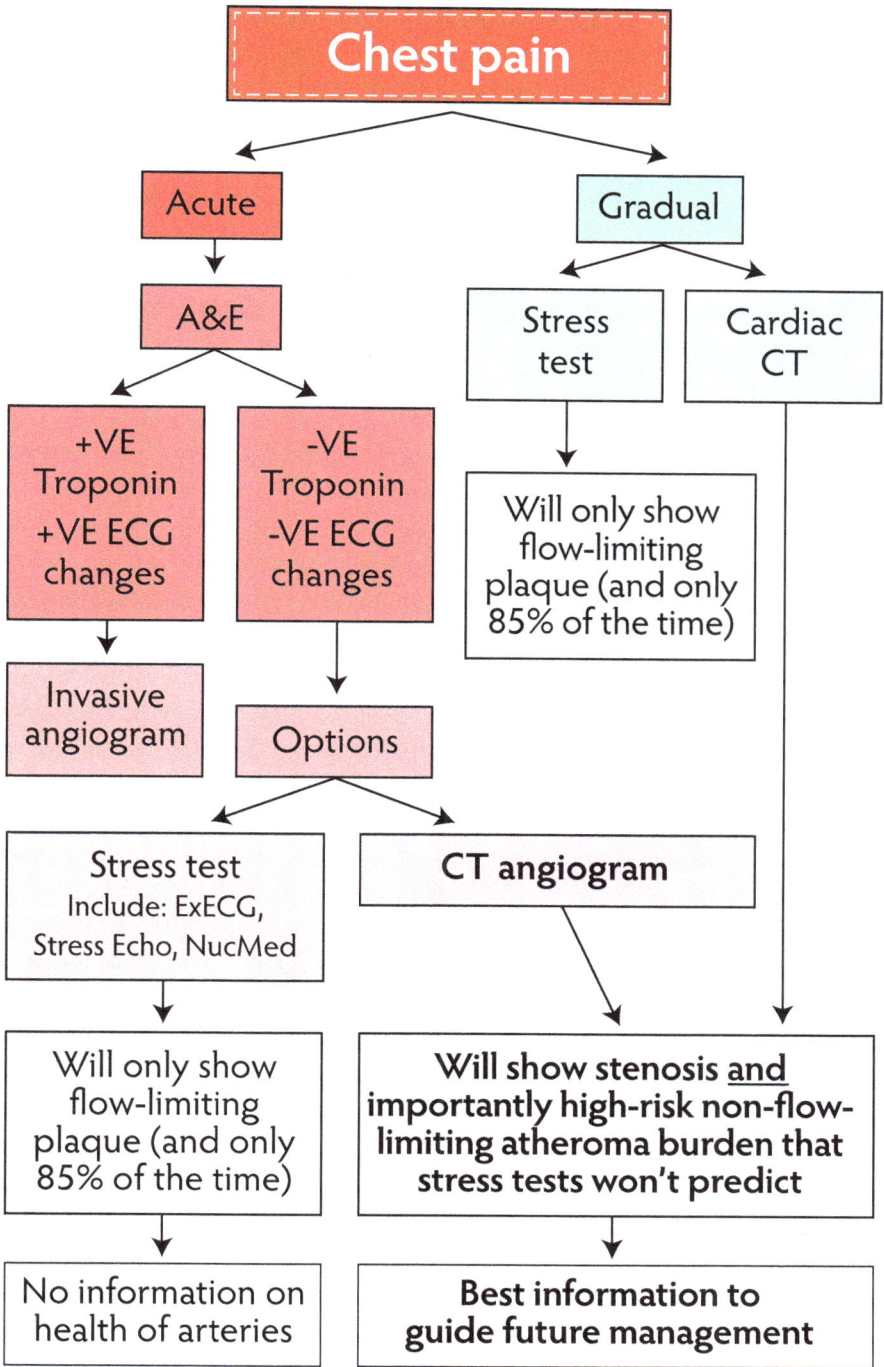

Chest pain

Acute
→ A&E
- +VE Troponin +VE ECG changes → Invasive angiogram
- -VE Troponin -VE ECG changes → Options
  - Stress test
    Include: ExECG, Stress Echo, NucMed
    → Will only show flow-limiting plaque (and only 85% of the time)
    → No information on health of arteries
  - **CT angiogram**
    → **Will show stenosis _and_ importantly high-risk non-flow-limiting atheroma burden that stress tests won't predict**
    → **Best information to guide future management**

Gradual
- Stress test
  → Will only show flow-limiting plaque (and only 85% of the time)
- Cardiac CT
  → **Will show stenosis _and_ importantly high-risk non-flow-limiting atheroma burden that stress tests won't predict**

I believe, however, that these two trials may have shown more of a benefit **for** the role of CCTA if they had been able to evaluate in more detail:

- that negative troponin/negative ECG patients of intermediate risk could be discharged home with aspirin, cholesterol agent and beta-blocker with a plan for urgent CT follow-up as an outpatient. This frees up the A&E service and reduces bed block.

- that the findings of non-flow-limiting atheroma burden defined by the cardiac CT test could then guide ongoing management of that individual patient into the future in the most precise way, remembering that this information would not be identified by stress testing.

- the role of knowing the *previous* cardiac CT information at time of presentation of an individual patient.

To highlight this, in my practice, I look to discharge patients from A&E who have no ECG changes and negative troponin, as the evidence suggests these patients carry a low risk. To ensure they carry an even lower risk until further evaluation, I start them on aspirin to keep their blood thin and on a cholesterol-lowering agent to stabilise any plaque that might be present. I will also commence beta-blockade to prevent rapid heart rate acceleration or significant blood pressure elevation, until we are able to evaluate them further.

Essentially I assume coronary artery disease until proven otherwise and start appropriate treatment. I am relying on the troponin to make sure these patients are not in immediate risk. I discharge them and look to an early, within at most 10 days, CT coronary angiogram to investigate for possible narrowings but also to evaluate for coronary atheroma burden in those patients who don't have narrowings. I will then see the patients to deal with the issues as found:

- If the cardiac CT scan shows no abnormality at all, I am happy to stop the medications, which the individual patient has been on only for a number of days with a very low risk of side-effects and at little cost. The reassurance of a 'clear scan' makes for an easier A&E evaluation should the patient present again with chest pain during the next few years (depending on specifics).

- If there is evidence from the cardiac CT scan that there may be a flow-limiting narrowing, and that it is clearly suggestive of a critical stenosis, the patient would have invasive coronary angiography with a view to an appropriate revascularisation strategy. The CT images will have prepared me for what to expect, for example, stent implantation.

- If the cardiac CT scan demonstrates the *possibility* of a narrowed lesion, then the patient would remain on the therapy implemented at the time of discharge from the A&E. I may put the person through treadmill testing to obtain a functional assessment of the possible narrowing as indicated on the cardiac CT. This would show if there were reduced flow to the heart muscle.

- If the cardiac CT scan does demonstrate the presence of atheroma burden but no suggestion of flow limitation, then I can make an evaluation to help the patient in future planning for his/her cardiovascular risk based on the C-PLUSS findings and other risk factors. This presents an opportunity to reduce future risk of event by implementation of appropriate therapy, which has been supported by observational (registry) data[7]. Therefore, the presentation to A&E has provided an opportunity to put in place appropriate prognostic management into the future for the individual.

Although this strategy is yet to be tested in trials, I have more than 25 cases (not a large number) all of which I have managed in this way, safely and in a timely fashion, without side-effects from the medication, or the occurrence of a MACE. (This is being submitted for publication, with the aim to follow up with a larger investigative study.) However, its components are all supported by evidence within the literature as referenced.

Patients are out of A&E more quickly and spend less time in hospital. For the patients who do not have a tight blockage, we are able to put in place risk stratification and be forewarned should those patients re-present to A&E in the future.

Also, by employing this strategy, I have significantly reduced my rates of invasive coronary angiography to find a diagnosis of 'normal coronary arteries'. This is important as the test is not only expensive but carries with it a risk of a major event, including stroke or heart attack, of between 1:1000 and 1:2000. I have available an audit, unpublished, from the main regional hospital in my area. This data[8] shows that up to 50 percent of first presentation A&E chest pain patients, who undergo invasive coronary angiography, have 'normal arteries'. In comparison, during the same period while I was employing the approach that I have described above, my own rate of normal arteries documented on first presentation chest pain ran at 15 percent[9]. This is supported by the SCOT-HEART trial, which demonstrated cardiac CT led to a significant reduction in the rates of patients progressing to invasive angiography[3].

This is a striking comparison, the significance of which lies in relation to the cost, which is enormous, as well as with the risk of side-effects, which is possible. It is important to remember, also, that invasive coronary angiography may show the inside of an artery looking normal, while cardiac CT imaging will show the wall of the artery, as well as the lumen of the artery, therefore, giving a better appreciation of health of that artery. The information gained from a normal invasive coronary angiogram is not as reassuring as that gained from cardiac CT imaging. For example, the images on the next page show an example of an invasive coronary angiogram reported as normal and the CCTA of the same patient.

Of course, in my suggested approach, there are situations in which the patient will have a cardiac CT scan, followed by invasive angiography. When this occurs, it means that the need for the expensive, invasive and risky test has been clearly established, based on the significance of the findings demonstrated on cardiac CT imaging; it has clearly been demonstrated to be the appropriate test.

Using the above cardiac CT guided approach, the imaging is cheaper, it is able to be done for the person as an outpatient and it has a risk profile that is nearly 100 times safer than invasive angiography. My experience has been that patients who progress from cardiac CT imaging to invasive coronary angiography are more than happy to have a safer test first to confirm that they really do need a more invasive and higher risk investigation.

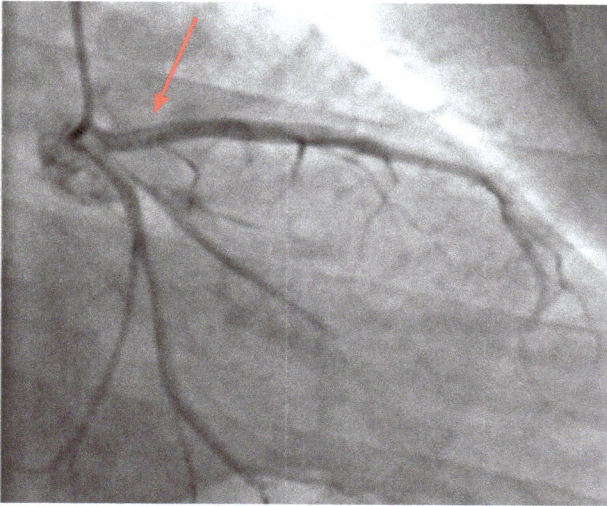

This is the invasive angiogram which reported the artery arrowed as "normal". The invasive angiogram is the gold standard for evaluating the anatomical features of narrowings or blockages.

The CT angiogram is excellent for showing us what might be going on in the wall of the artery **before** a blockage develops.

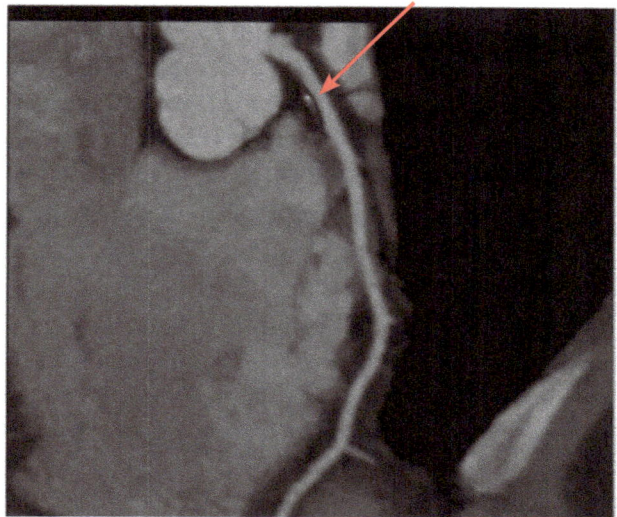

This is the same patient with the arrow marking where there is a high-risk plaque, which at this stage had not encroached on the lumen (the inside) of the artery.

CCS and chest pain

In this chapter on evaluation of chest pain, I have not suggested the use of a zero calcium score as a gatekeeper to CCTA as I did in the chapter on risk. This is because, in the evaluation of calcium score for chest pain, Schenker et.al demonstrated a rate of MACE of nearly four percent per annum[10] in the patients with a zero CCS. This suggests that in the situation of chest pain presentation, calcium score alone does not provide enough information to deal with possible flow-limiting coronary artery disease. This makes sense if we think of the group of patients who may have high-risk atheroma burden greater than suggested by their calcium score alone[11].

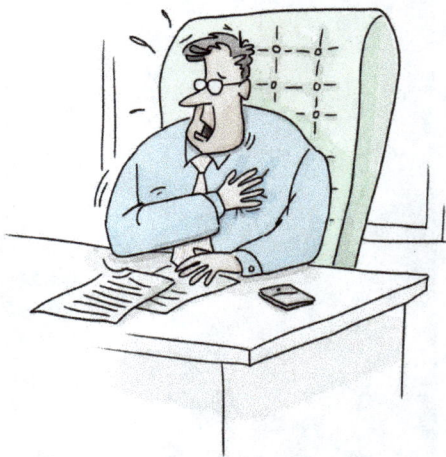

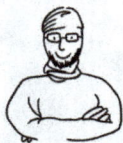

My hope is that, in the future, there will be a randomised controlled trial looking at the approach that I employ for A&E chest pain presentation. My data suggests that it is safe and effective. However, I have not been randomising patients. Safety and benefit need to be clearly demonstrated.

My other hope is that if this approach is proven safe, then it could be implemented by a regional health body, with close assessment given to provide data on cost and outcome.

Until this approach is studied, evaluated and published, it will not be widely appreciated and utilised. However, I believe it is important to open discussion around this method which appears safe for the patient, and economical for both the patient and the community.

- Not all chest pain that presents to Accident and Emergency will be the heart.

- Not all chest pain that presents to Accident and Emergency will put the person in hospital.

- A blood test called troponin, if negative, together with ECG features that do not change, can suggest the patient is at low risk of an event within 30 days. My practice is to give these patients medication to reduce even further the risk of having a cardiac event and to bring them back as outpatients in an expedient fashion to evaluate and treat, as indicated by the results of these tests.

- Such an approach presents an opportunity to reduce costs to hospitals and to reduce the amount of invasive testing for patients. This, in turn, reduces costs and minimises complications.

- The unique value of a cardiac CT strategy is that it will demonstrate two situations that cannot be identified any other way:

  » high risk atheroma burden without flow limitation that carries a high risk and would not show on a stress test or an invasive angiogram, and

  » no or low-risk atheroma burden which allows clear guidance for appropriate care for that patient over the next 5 to 10 years.

- By utilising the cardiac CT approach, a chest pain presentation can become an opportunity to be best informed to manage that patient for the next 5 to 10 years.

[1]   Anderson JL, Adams CD, Antman EM, et al. ACC/AHA 2007 guidelines for the management of patients with unstable angina/non-ST-Elevation myocardial infarction: a report of the American College of Cardiology/American Heart Association Task Force on Practice Guidelines (Writing Committee to Revise the 2002 Guidelines for the Management of Patients With Unstable Angina/Non-ST Elevation Myocardial Infarction) developed in collaboration with the American College of Emergency Physicians, the Society for Cardiovascular Angiography and

Interventions, and the Society of Thoracic Surgeons endorsed by the American Association of Cardiovascular and Pulmonary Rehabilitation and the Society for Academic Emergency Medicine. J Am Coll Cardiol 2007;50:e1-e157.

[2]   Douglas PS, Hoffmann U, Lee KL, et al. PROspective Multicenter Imaging Study for Evaluation of chest pain: rationale and design of the PROMISE trial. Am Heart J 2014;167:796-803.e1.

[3]   CT coronary angiography in patients with suspected angina due to coronary heart disease (SCOT-HEART): an open-label, parallel-group, multicentre trial. The Lancet;385:2383-91.

[4]   Hoffmann U, Bamberg F, Chae CU, et al. Coronary computed tomography angiography for early triage of patients with acute chest pain: the ROMICAT (Rule Out Myocardial Infarction using Computer Assisted Tomography) trial. J Am Coll Cardiol 2009;53:1642-50.

[5]   Hulten E, Goehler A, Bittencourt MS, et al. Cost and resource utilization associated with use of computed tomography to evaluate chest pain in the emergency department: the Rule Out Myocardial Infarction using Computer Assisted Tomography (ROMICAT) study. Circulation Cardiovascular quality and outcomes 2013;6:514-24.

[6]   Galperin-Aizenberg M, Cook TS, Hollander JE, Litt HI. Cardiac CT Angiography in the Emergency Department. American Journal of Roentgenology 2015;204:463-74.

[7]   Chow BJW, Small G, Yam Y, et al. Prognostic and Therapeutic Implications of Statin and Aspirin Therapy in Individuals With Nonobstructive Coronary Artery Disease: Results From the CONFIRM (Coronary CT Angiography Evaluation For Clinical Outcomes: An International Multicenter Registry) Registry. Arterioscler Thromb Vasc Biol 2015;35:981-89.

[8]   Costello B, (2012). CATH LAB AUDIT RHH 2012, Raw Data

[9]   Bishop W, PRACTICE AUDIT (2014). Cardiac CT, Unpublished Data

[10]   Schenker MP, Dorbala S, Hong EC, et al. Interrelation of coronary calcification, myocardial ischemia, and outcomes in patients with intermediate likelihood of coronary artery disease: a combined positron emission tomography/computed tomography study. Circulation 2008;117:1693-700.

[11]   Naya M, Murthy VL, Foster CR, et al. Prognostic Interplay of Coronary Artery Calcification and Underlying Vascular Dysfunction in Patients With Suspected Coronary Artery Disease. J Am Coll Cardiol 2013;61:2098-106.

Reducing the likelihood of sudden cardiac death is considered in the next chapter.

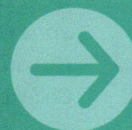

Chapter 14 -
Managing symptoms and prognosis

> managing symptoms and prognosis:
  – living as well as possible for as long as possible

If a patient has symptoms from a build-up of cholesterol in the arteries causing a narrowing, or if the patient shows a significant atheroma burden on cardiac CT but no symptoms to that stage, the approach for management shares several basic principles.

In the first instance, our hope is to reduce the likelihood of sudden cardiac death. This is achieved by reducing the possibility of a clot suddenly forming within the artery at the site of a ruptured plaque. Whether there is a narrowing atherosclerotic plaque or an early atherosclerotic plaque causing no flow limitation, both situations can give rise to the splitting of the covering cap of the cholesterol plaque. This fissuring allows the contents of the blood to come into contact with the contents of the plaque. It is the meeting of these substances that leads to a clot forming within the artery. Autopsy data of patients who have experienced the sudden formation of a clot in their arteries, and have subsequently died, show that over 50 percent of acute myocardial infarctions occur in arteries that have a plaque that is narrowing the lumen by greater than 70 percent. That means that almost 50 percent are occurring on arteries that are non-flow-limiting and therefore causing no symptoms[1-3] prior to an event.

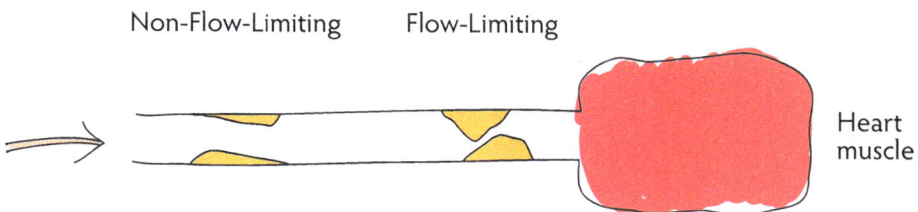

Non-Flow-Limiting   Flow-Limiting   Heart muscle

If we were to section through these plaques, both narrowed and non-narrowed, we would find similar features. We would see the lumen (inside space) of the artery, the cholesterol build-up and a fibrous cap over the cholesterol build-up. This occurs in both situations which is why both can cause plaque rupture and sudden cardiac death. It is a plaque rupture causing sudden cardiac death when the plaque was non-flow-limiting that gives rise to an all-too-common situation, that of an otherwise fit and well person dying, without warning, prematurely, from a heart attack.

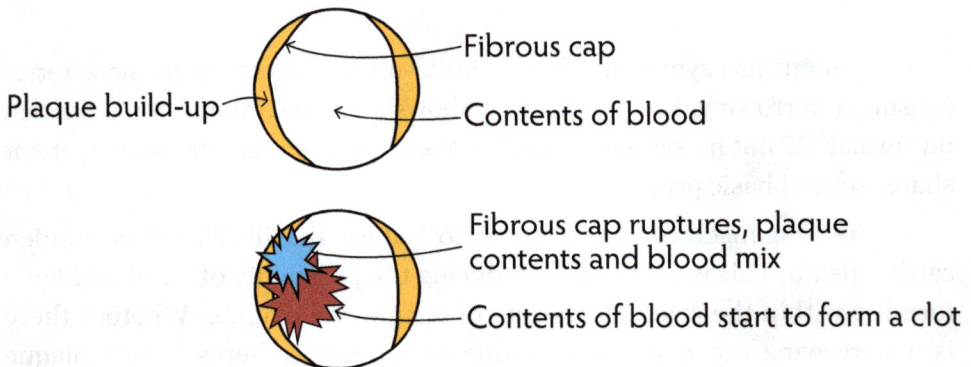

Plaque build-up ——— Fibrous cap

——— Contents of blood

Fibrous cap ruptures, plaque contents and blood mix

——— Contents of blood start to form a clot

There are several areas that we can address to stabilise this process.

- **We can reduce the stickiness of the platelets** which reduces the likelihood of a clot developing. This is done using aspirin or aspirin-like agents; these are called anti-platelets.

- **We can stabilise the plaque** by reducing its vulnerability and altering its components so that it is less likely to contain soft, unstable, cholesterol-dominant lipids or fats. To do this we use the statin agents. *(It is possible that the statin agents offer benefits beyond lowering the cholesterol. They may contribute to reducing inflammation within the plaque. That data is not robust but is certainly interesting.)*

- **We can reduce the stress and strain on the fibrous plaque** by reducing blood pressure and attending to life-style issues, such as smoking, exercise and appropriate eating.

When it comes to how we deal with coronary atheroma or coronary artery disease, there are really only two criteria on which we focus and there are three interventions available.

Essentially we aim to have people:

- **live as well as possible, for as long as possible.** Or put another way, we aim to minimise symptoms and maximise prognosis.

The three major interventions are:

- **medicines/drugs** such as aspirin, statins and anti-anginals (the drugs used to reduce or treat angina);
- **balloons** or **stents** (an intravascular device deployed percutaneously, through the skin), and
- coronary artery **bypass grafting** (major surgery that allows a 'bypassing' of the diseased section of artery by using an alternate vessel, generally from the aorta, to supply blood to the heart).

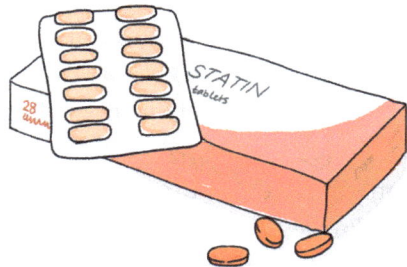

Management	Symptoms	Prognosis
MEDICINES Asprin (and similar) Statins (and similar) Anti-anginals	Good for a fair number of patients (Perhaps suitable for 50+%) ★★☆	Essential for all situations to stabilise plaque and reduce progression ★★★
STENTS OR BALLOONS	Very good for localised narrowing ★★★	Evidence for stenting or ballooning for prognosis limited to a few studies ★
SURGERY Coronary artery bypass grafting	May not be able to graft all affected arteries and recovery can be significant ★★☆	For the sickest patients with poorly functioning hearts; if they can survive, it is very good prognostically ★★★

MEDICINES When it comes to medicines and managing the symptoms, we find that in a reasonable number of patients, medications do an adequate job. They are effective in, perhaps, two-thirds of patients, thus allowing a conservative approach for a significant number of people. When it comes to medicines and prognosis, there is no question that medicines form the foundation of our management to modify risk into the future. Thinning the blood using aspirin or aspirin-like agents, minimising progression of and stabilising plaque formation by the use of statins or other cholesterol-lowering agents, and treatment of blood pressure and other risk factors are absolutely central to modification of future risk and, therefore, are the mainstay of any prognostic intervention.

BALLOONS or STENTS The implantation of a stent can be extremely effective at symptom management when there is a single isolated narrowing that has the characteristics to allow a stent to be inserted. When we consider stenting in terms of *prognostic* management, the data is not quite so solid. A stent placed to unblock the narrowed portion of artery does not necessarily deal with the non-flow-limiting plaque that could be elsewhere in the coronary tree which may still subsequently progress and lead to problems. However, using a stent improves the outcome when it restores normal flow to a large area of heart muscle. This was suggested by a subset assessment of a study called the Courage Trial[4]. This is a simple concept: if the fuel line to one cylinder of your V8 engine (12.5 percent) is a bit blocked, the car may still be okay but if two cylinders are affected (25 percent), then the engine will not run well and it ought to be fixed.

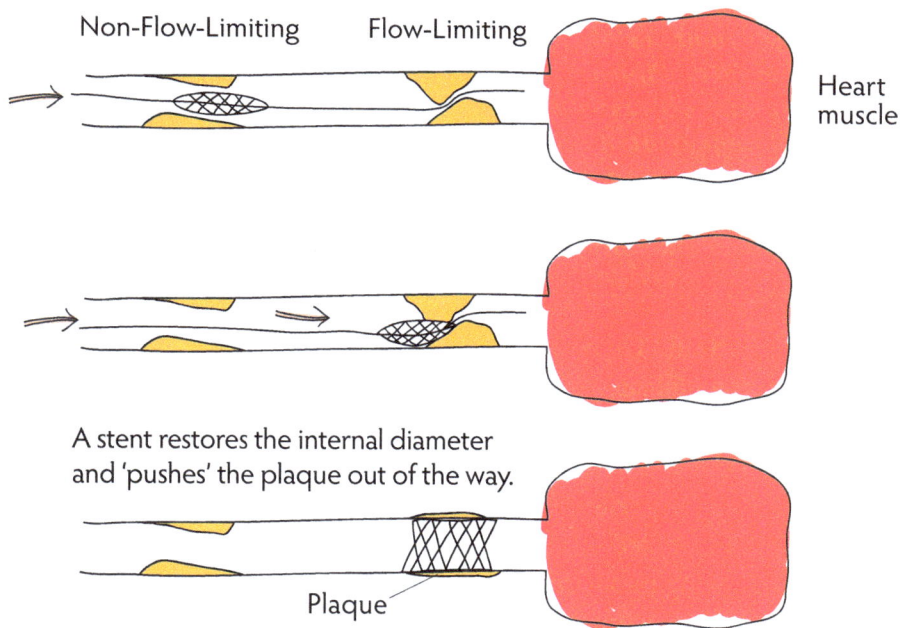

Stent implantation restores flow at the site of focal narrowing. However, it does not address non-flow-limiting plaque.

SURGERY From a symptomatic point of view, surgery can be extremely good in appropriately selected patients. These are people who have extensive coronary artery disease which is too complex to be addressed with stenting alone and for whom medication has not been successful. These patients will describe significant improvement in their symptoms after surgery, although the surgery is not without risk and has a significant convalescent period. When it comes to surgery and *prognosis,* there is no question that patients who have the sickest hearts (if they can be managed through the surgical process and survive) will do better than not having had the surgery. Generally, the decision to operate is taken on the grounds that a large amount of poorly working heart muscle can be resupplied with blood. The risks of the surgery are outweighed by the potential benefits of restoring the blood flow to large parts of the heart muscle.

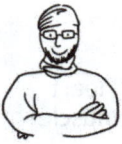

It is important to understand that, as a profession, we consider the extent of shortage of blood flow to the heart in a prognostic way. The Courage Trial (which looked at an intervention [stents] versus conservative approach [medication] in the management of coronary artery disease) certainly suggested that, if an area of heart exceeding 15 percent of the total left ventricular myocardium were receiving inadequate blood flow, then restoration of that blood flow would improve the outlook for that patient.

This is important. There will be times when a patient potentially has a narrowing in a smallish vessel in a distal location. On stress testing, the patient may perform extremely well with little evidence that a major area of heart muscle has been affected. This patient would, based on what we understand, be appropriately managed conservatively, particularly if the patient were not troubled by symptoms. In contrast, if a patient were to have an area of narrowing in one of the large arteries which supplied a significant amount of the myocardium, and a stress test showed a substantial area of heart muscle affected by lack of flow, then current evidence suggests that that person would benefit from having revascularisation (re-establishment of blood flow), either by angioplasty (unblocking the artery) or by coronary artery bypass grafting, depending on what was technically appropriate.

IMPORTANT POINTS ✔

- Treatment has two main objectives: symptoms and prognosis. We want people to live as well as possible, for as long as possible.

- We have at our means medicines, stents/balloons and coronary bypass grafting. The use of these options is guided by the individual needs of the patient but in every circumstance, prognostic management will include some sort of medicine + lifestyle modification.

- Re-establishing the blood flow by balloons, stents or bypass grafting becomes more likely the greater the amount of heart that is affected by impeded blood flow through a narrowed artery.

[1] Ambrose JA, Tannenbaum MA, Alexopoulos D, et al. Angiographic progression of coronary artery disease and the development of myocardial infarction. J Am Coll Cardiol 1988;12:56-62.

[2] Giroud D, Li JM, Urban P, Meier B, Rutishauer W. Relation of the site of acute myocardial infarction to the most severe coronary arterial stenosis at prior angiography. Am J Cardiol 1992;69:729-32.

[3] Little WC, Constantinescu M, Applegate RJ, et al. Can coronary angiography predict the site of a subsequent myocardial infarction in patients with mild-to moderate coronary artery disease? Circulation 1988;78:1157-66.

[4] Shaw LJ, Berman DS, Maron DJ, et al. Optimal Medical Therapy With or Without Percutaneous Coronary Intervention to Reduce Ischemic Burden: Results From the Clinical Outcomes Utilizing Revascularization and Aggressive Drug Evaluation (COURAGE) Trial Nuclear Substudy. Circulation 2008;117:1283-91.

In the next chapter, chance findings can be hugely beneficial to a patient but, before that, we discuss an important side-issue, the risk of stroke. →

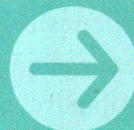

what is my risk of a stroke?

Many of the patients who come to see me about their risk of heart attack are also concerned about their risk of stroke.

A heart attack is the term for a major adverse coronary event, or a blockage or partial blockage of a coronary, or **heart,** artery. A stroke is the sudden blockage or partial blockage of a blood vessel supplying the **brain.**

This can occur in the same way as in the coronary arteries: with ruptured plaque and formation of a clot or thrombus. If this occurs in the arteries leading to the brain, the carotid arteries of the neck, then often the clot will break off and travel to the brain circulation and lodge in a vessel causing lack of blood supply beyond that point. This is call a 'thrombo-embolic' stroke (*embolic* means carried through the blood stream).

Plaque can also form within the arteries that supply the brain. In this situation, if a plaque ruptures and a clot forms at that site (as happens in the coronary arteries), this is called a 'thrombotic' stroke.

Both thrombo-embolic and thrombotic stroke risk are managed the same way as coronary atheroma: with aspirin, statins and related risk factor modification, blood pressure management, treatment of diabetes and lifestyle modifications, including cessation of smoking.

This means that if the cardiac CT findings are such that risk modification with medication and lifestyle intervention are indicated, this will also reduce the risk of stroke.

What is not so clear from the literature is this: *If there is a zero or low coronary calcium score, does this indicate the patient has a zero or low risk of stroke?*

This is important as one could make a decision not to treat based on the cardiac findings and leave the patient at risk of stroke, if there were atheroma burden within the carotid arteries or the cerebral arteries. In general terms, the suggestion from the literature is that the coronary vessels are the ones that demonstrate the most wear and tear because of the movement of the heart. If there is significant atheroma burden in the heart, then there is a good chance it will be in the cerebral (brain-related) circulation also. The opposite is also suggested: if the heart is clear, the cerebral vessels are probably also clear[1].

In my own practice, in certain situations, I will organise carotid ultrasound imaging before making a decision on withholding the use of aspirin and statins long-term for an individual who has a zero coronary calcium score but who may have some other risk factors, such as elevated cholesterol or hypertension. These could mean the person has a risk of stroke not reflected by the state of the coronary arteries. Until the data is clearer, I think this is a reasonable way forward.

It is important to know, too, that there are several other types of stroke.

Stroke can also occur from a rupture of a blood vessel in the brain, leading to bleeding into the brain. This is called a haemorrhagic stroke and is often related to elevated blood pressure levels and sometimes defects within the artery wall.

The other important and common type of stroke is from atrial fibrillation. Atrial fibrillation is a condition in which the chambers of the 'top part of the heart', the chambers that receive blood from the body or from the lungs *(see Chapter 1)* lose their electrical synchronicity and have a discordant, irregular, random electrical rhythm. This leads, essentially, to failure of the atria to contract, with the subsequent pooling and stasis, or inactivity of blood, within the atrium. When the blood pools, it may form a clot in one of the recesses of the left atrium. If a clot forms, it may break free and travel to the brain, lodging in an artery and leading to stroke. Assessment of the risk of cerebral haemorrhage and atrial fibrillation with embolism from the heart are beyond the scope of this book but are important issues to discuss with your doctor.

[1]   Budoff MJ, Hokanson JE, Nasir K, et al. Progression of coronary artery calcium predicts all-cause mortality. JACC: Cardiovascular Imaging 2010;3:1229-36.

Testimonial

I am a 62-year-old female who has had very high cholesterol for the past 15 years. I have refused cholesterol-lowing drugs due to a reaction I had to one eight years ago. I have never smoked and there is no heart disease in my family. I also suffer with polymyalgia which is an inflammation of the muscles. Thus my fear of taking statins.

Recently my GP suggested that I at least go through testing of my heart arteries with Dr Warrick Bishop, a cardiac specialist, to put my mind at rest. Not all patients who have high cholesterol have plaque on their arteries. Unfortunately, I wasn't one of those patients. However, I would highly recommend having the test done. I now have life choices to make to assist in preventing a heart attack in the future. Had I not had the testing done, l might have just not woken up one day, like a friend of mine. She had not undergone any testing. One morning she woke up feeling unwell. Having decided to lie on the couch for a while, her husband found her gone at 10am. She was 69. This sort of testing also gives your children life choices for preventative measures much earlier, if they choose to follow that path.

Susanne Dart

Chapter 15 -
Chance findings

> incidental findings that are not predictable but can be very beneficial

In medicine, 'incidental findings' are those discoveries made by chance that may or may not be beneficial to the patient. There are a couple of situations that I have seen in clinical presentations which warrant consideration:

1) calcium seen in the heart during a chest CT scan undertaken for another reason, and

2) non-cardiac findings during a cardiac CT.

Finding calcium in the heart through a non-cardiac scan

I recently was asked to see Pamela, a 63-year-old, who had suffered several weeks of rib pain. While investigating this, her doctor had ordered a CT of the chest wall. This showed no significant abnormality of the chest wall or untoward cause of her pain but it was noted that she had calcium in her heart.

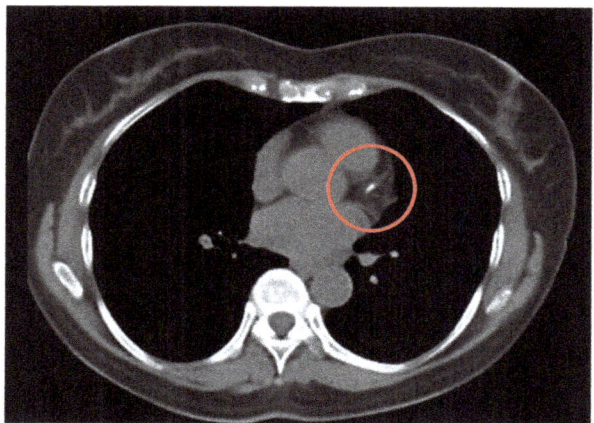

A CT of the chest wall picks up calcium in Pam's heart.

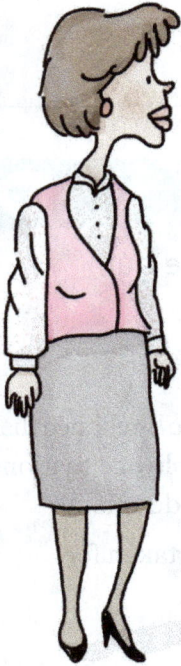

There was not a lot, as suggested by the image. The patient was otherwise well and had no symptoms attributable to the heart. She and her husband were due to leave on a six-week trip to Europe within a few weeks. We spoke at some length about the pros and cons of imaging. Pamela, in consultation with her husband, decided she wanted more information. *If there were no problem, great; if there were a problem, then let's deal with it.* So, they paid for a cardiac scan.

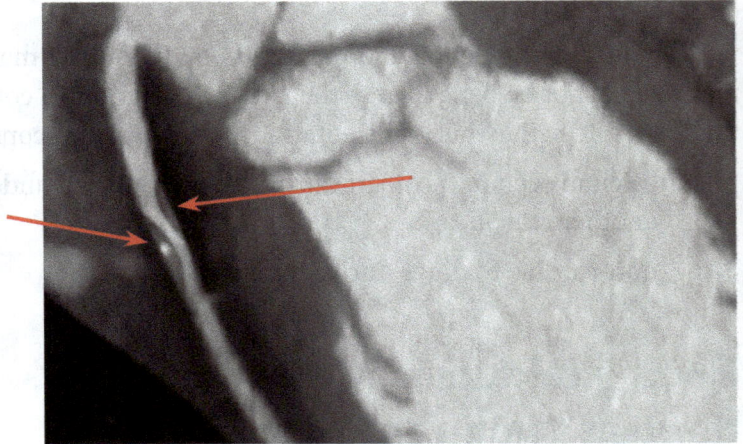

The resulting image *(above)* showed a small amount of calcium associated with a significant amount of non-calcific plaque, resulting in narrowing of the artery of approximately 50 percent. The features of this plaque are considered high-risk of an event in the next five to 10 years. The use of aspirin and cholesterol-lowering medication would reduce risk and improve the outcome.

Interestingly, this was the *only* plaque that Pam had in her entire coronary tree but importantly, the plaque was in the beginning section of a major artery and, if it blocked, would have disastrous consequences.

Pam's blood pressure was normal, her cholesterol profile was unremarkable and based on current Australian guidelines, she did not qualify for the subsidised prescription of statins. She and her husband were more than happy to have the information. They elected to pay for the statin therapy (we halved cost by prescribing the highest dose, of 80mg, with her taking half a tablet, 40mg, thus achieving the target LDL levels for her) and aspirin. Their trip overseas went without problems; the medication is well tolerated and she is well educated and aware that **any** suspicious symptoms warrant immediate medical review.

No one can say where the alternative road would have led. However, in this case Pam and her husband were able to have as much information as possible, with pros and cons explained, and they were able to make a decision that *they* were comfortable with, looking to the future.

Although it might seem obvious to use the incidental finding of calcium in the heart to help guide best patient management, there are limitations. Because the heart moves with each beat, the non-cardiac scans may show blurring and provide inaccurate calcium appreciation. There is no standard for reporting the heart in non-cardiac scans, so in some situations, calcium will be reported and in other situations not, based on reporter preference[1,2]. In time, guidelines will be formulated. Now, however, patients should be aware that **if they have a CT scan of the chest they could also ask if the scan detected calcium in the heart.**

Finding something else during a cardiac scan

When a patient is sent for a cardiac scan, together with the findings relating to the heart, something else of seeming significance can be found in up to 40 percent of cases. Importantly, and fortunately for the patient, however, fewer than five percent of extra-cardiac findings have prognostic significance[3].

When Mike came to see me he was in his mid-to-late 60s. He had shortness of breath and in the work-up, I felt that cardiac CT imaging would help in diagnosis and management.

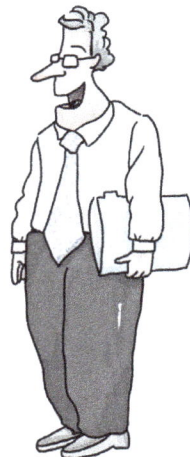

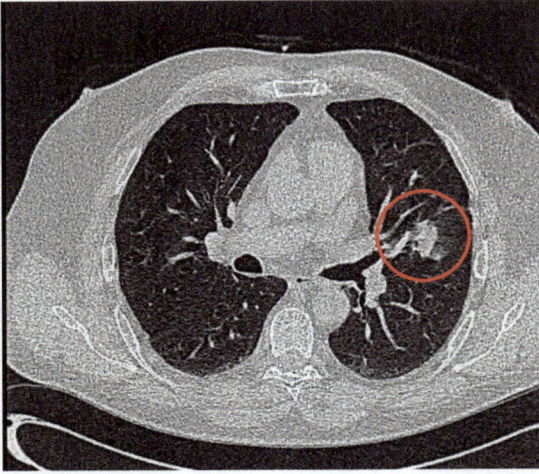

Here is Mike's CCTA result. The circle highlights a nodular soft tissue mass. This was seen by the radiologist reviewing the study and was described in the final report.

Mike went on to further imaging and evaluation, and was diagnosed with lung cancer. He underwent surgery which went well. When I saw him last, he was two years post-surgery and his cancer doctor had given him the all clear.

He did have plaque in his arteries and we also dealt with this.

This was just lucky for Mike. His outlook, had the cancer not been found when it was, would certainly have been very different.

Both these situations were purely chance findings. They presented situations we could not predict but could take advantage of, for the benefit of the patient.

Sometimes, a chance finding may lead to further investigation(s) which could be costly or may even carry risk-without-benefit to the patient. There is no clear cut answer to this. However, I decide on further testing based on the clinical situation, the specifics of the chance finding, the most appropriate further testing and discussion with the patient. There is no right or wrong, just the most sensible way forward given a particular situation.

IMPORTANT POINT ☑

- There is no right or wrong about chance findings. Sometimes they can be very advantageous. Each instance must be determined on its own merit, in the clinical context and in consultation with the patient.

[1]   *White CS, Jerome S. Coronary calcium scoring on nongated chest CT: Is it ready for prime time? Journal of cardiovascular computed tomography;5:119-21.*

[2]   *White CS, Jerome S. Coronary calcium scoring on nongated chest CT: Is it ready for prime time? Journal of cardiovascular computed tomography;5:119-21.*

[3]   *Karius P, Schuetz GM, Schlattmann P, Dewey M. Extracardiac findings on coronary CT angiography: A systematic review. Journal of cardiovascular computed tomography;8:174-82.e6.*

Any change brings with it potential threat. In the next chapter we look at some reasons why the system is resistant to change. →

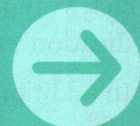

Case histories - Tony and Heather McKenny

Both are retired professionals, fit and presenting with no obvious symptoms of heart disease.

HEATHER – AGED 67

Heather has no known family history of high cholesterol and would have a very low score on any cardiovascular disease risk assessment chart. In particular, her cholesterol readings were always very low. Despite having been made aware through a public lecture at her local gym that these factors did not necessarily preclude the risk of calcification, she decided that a CT scan was not necessary.

However, sometime later following a CT chest scan after a persistent cough, one of the radiology findings mentioned some coronary artery calcification. Her GP referred her to me. I found her CT coronary angiography demonstrated significant plaque in just one particular spot which, if left unattended, posed a high to very high health risk. Treatment, in the form of statin medication and aspirin, was started immediately.

Had this CT scan not been taken she would have felt protected by her good cholesterol readings and healthy life style, while unwittingly, actually being at significant risk of a heart attack at any time.

TONY – AGED 69

Tony, on the other hand, has a long family history of high cholesterol levels and heart disease, and has been on statin medication for some years. However, other than a high cholesterol level, Tony is fit and would appear to have a very low risk of cardiovascular disease against any commonly used assessment tool.

Following the gym talk, he arranged for a check-up to see if there were evidence of plaque deposition in the arteries. The CT scan showed there was, in fact, very little evidence of plaque deposits and he was able to tailor his medication to further control the cholesterol at an appropriate level.

In addition, the cardiac CT angiography has provided an important base-line measure for future monitoring of the health of his arteries.

Chapter 16 -
Hurdles to change

> why there has been a slow up-take

Throughout the book, I have written about the concept of cardiac CT imaging which combines both coronary calcium scoring with coronary angiography. I have specifically used the term 'cardiac CT' to describe the process that allows not only anatomical assessment of the heart but also prognostic assessment. I have also outlined how I think the information obtained can help the clinician best manage the needs of an individual patient.

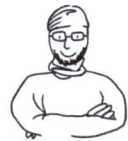

WELL, WHY IS THIS NOT BEING DONE ON A REGULAR BASIS?
Is what I am suggesting so left-field that it is potentially out of the realm of current medical therapy? Am I bordering on alternative medicine practices?

I don't believe so. I would like to offer several points for consideration.

No evidence base for support

FIRSTLY, and I have said this several times already, **there are no double-blind randomised controlled trials** supporting what I have described when using cardiac CT imaging for risk stratification. There is no question that should those trials be available, they would be a valuable asset to the care of individuals. The reality, however, is that it is quite possible these studies will never happen for the very reason that they would need to define high-risk individuals who would then be randomised to treatment or not.

As an example, let's consider that we look to study the use of cardiac CT imaging to improve outcomes in a risk management situation. In the trial that we are going to run, we will take one hundred 50-year-old men who, by standard Framingham-style risk calculators, have a 15 percent chance of an event in 10 years.

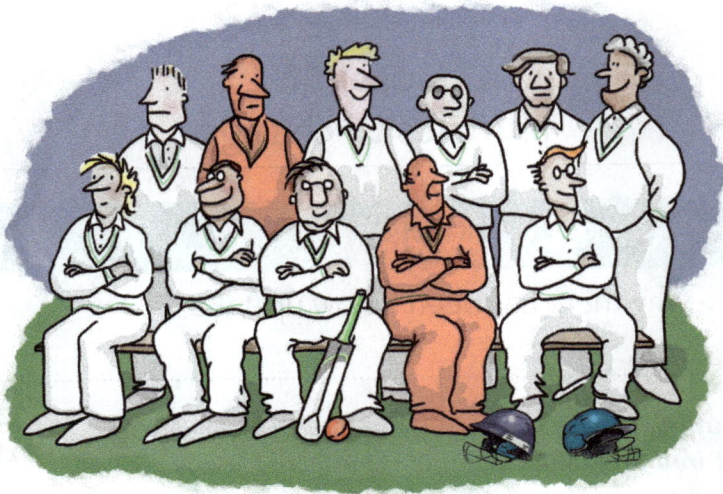

To put the proposed trial scenario into a more relatable context: if we took an 11-man cricket team, all 50 years of age, on these numbers one to two of those men would have a MACE within 10 years.

We know that the population of 100 intermediate-risk men will demonstrate features of a population distribution. That means that most of the population will be intermediate risk but there will be outliers at each end of the group who will have a much lower or much higher risk.

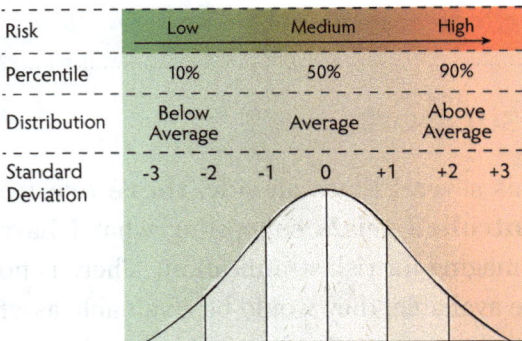

Risk	Low	Medium	High
Percentile	10%	50%	90%
Distribution	Below Average	Average	Above Average
Standard Deviation	-3 -2 -1	0 +1	+2 +3

We will scan those patients using cardiac CT. We will likely find between 10 and 20 of those individuals who have high-risk features, suggesting that they would be the individuals likely to have an event over the 10 year observational period. Having found the high-risk patients, we then invite them to take part in the study where, for half of them, we initiate treatment which we know will reduce risk in a primary preventative role and, for the other half, we invite them to take a placebo and see what happens.

Let me ask you: If you had a 50:50 chance of being in the placebo group, how comfortable would you feel about this study? If you were the doctor, would you enrol patients? Further, if you were a member of an ethics committee evaluating this study, how comfortable would you feel about potentially sacrificing the 7 to 10 patients per 100 (or 70-100 per 1000) found to be at high risk but not offered treatment, just to prove what happens?

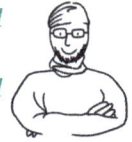

Herein lies a dilemma of evidence-based medicine.

The data around the use of cardiac CT imaging for risk is patchy and, in some ways, has led us in the wrong direction. Earlier, I mentioned the St Francis Heart Trial[1]. This was to be the trial that would prove that CCS-guided treatment would lead to improved outcomes. Unfortunately, it didn't.

The researchers took just over 1000 asymptomatic subjects who had CCS at or above the 80th percentile for age and sex, and randomised them to statin therapy, plus anti-oxidant vitamins at the onset of the study, which lasted about four and a half years. That means half received treatment; the other half didn't. The intent was to see if there would be a reduction in MACE in the treatment group.

The study had a few problems.

- The ethics of the day dictated that if any calcium were detected, then the subject should be on aspirin, whether that person was in the treatment **or** placebo group. A safe thing for the participants but it immediately diminished the likelihood of a statistical difference between the treatment arm and the non-treatment arm. In this study, **the control arm was treated with aspirin.**

- The dose of cholesterol treatment selected was 20mg of atorvastatin. This is a relatively low dose and probably less than I would select for someone who is at or above the 80th percentile for age and sex. It is possible **the intervention group was under-treated.**

- Twenty-five percent of the patients were female and some of these were under 60 years of age. Twenty-five percent had a CCS under 150, suggesting an approximate six percent risk of an event in 10 years but, because of the score being at or above the 80th percentile, an increased lifetime risk. Remember that as the study only went for just over four years, it is likely **it just didn't run for long enough for these intermediate-risk patients to have an event.**

These factors mean the study was almost doomed to fail. Participants of the control (non-treatment) group were given treatment (aspirin). The treatment group was probably under-treated. There were a number of subjects who were not likely to have a problem within the study period (low absolute score with high percentile, so representing low to intermediate risk with increased lifetime risk) so that there were not enough events to come to a meaningful conclusion. It is interesting to note that when they looked more closely at the spread of coronary calcium scores, there was a strong suggestion that the intervention was beneficial in the group of patients with scores above 400, the ones with the highest absolute risk. However, they just didn't have enough numbers to draw this as a final conclusion to the trial. Also, they found a reduction in MACE from 9.9 percent to 6.9 percent over a fairly short follow-up period, although the study was underpowered to show a statistical difference.

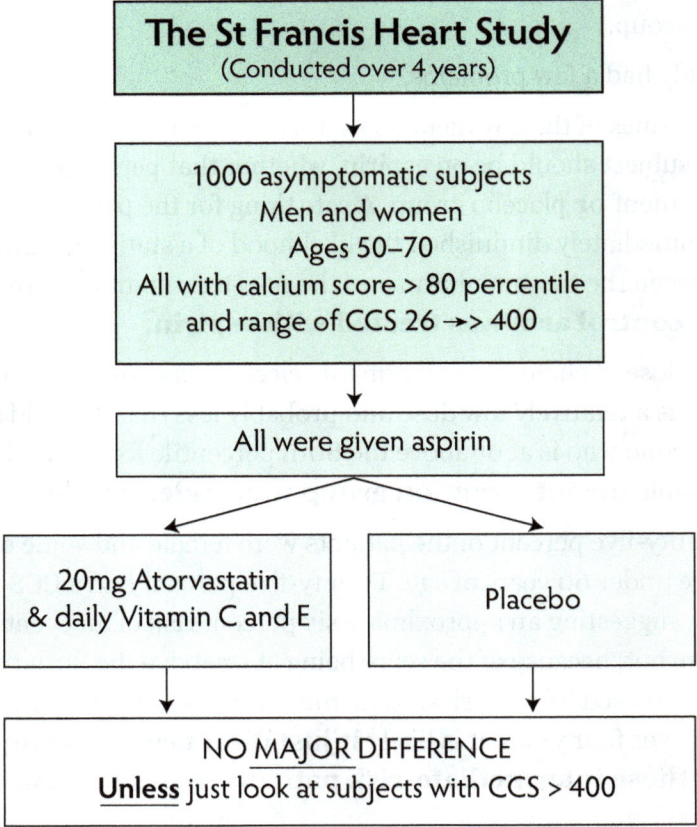

The St Francis Heart Study
(Conducted over 4 years)

↓

1000 asymptomatic subjects
Men and women
Ages 50–70
All with calcium score > 80 percentile
and range of CCS 26 –→> 400

↓

All were given aspirin

20mg Atorvastatin
& daily Vitamin C and E

Placebo

NO MAJOR DIFFERENCE
Unless just look at subjects with CCS > 400

I'm pretty sure I wouldn't be writing this book if they had selected patients with scores above 400, used 80mg of atorvastatin, hadn't treated the control arm with aspirin and had run the trial for 10 years – *but I can't prove that!*

The reality is that the randomised controlled data for using cardiac CT in the way I have proposed will likely never exist. When the alternative is to randomise individuals at high risk of MACE without treatment, which is unpalatable on many levels, we can only ever hope to obtain robust longitudinal observational data, watching over time to see how something works.

In this situation, does the lack of data mean that we should not use the information that appears implied from what is available? To my way of thinking, the Parachute Study *(see page 67)* answers that question. I also believe that we have an obligation to use what we feel to be most appropriate in a given patient's situation for that person's well being if, from a clinical perspective, we believe that the available evidence suggests it is the right course of action for that person.

Different disciplines, different bias

SECONDLY, cardiac CT falls within several disciplines and is represented with a slightly different bias in different arenas.

Radiologists, by virtue of their proximity to CT scanners, were significantly involved in the development of the technology and are, by training, focussed predominantly on the accuracy of anatomy. Many of the studies on the role of coronary angiography have been anatomically driven to look at the role of the technology to complement, or sometimes replace, invasive coronary angiography, which is also an anatomical test. There is no question that the anatomy is important. There is no question that CT coronary angiography has been validated in providing reproducible and robust data in evaluation of anatomical issues surrounding the heart[2,3]. This focus on anatomical validation has taken the spotlight, such that prognostic validation has fallen into a blind spot.

Cardiologists working in the area of risk stratification early in the development of scanning of the heart, doctors such as Agatston, used calcium

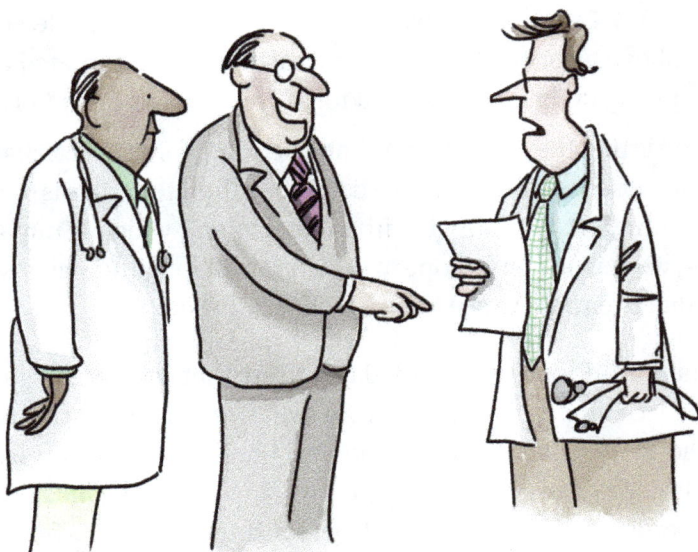

The patient's best interests are served by bringing together the experience and expertise of the three disciplines.

as an indicator to help guide risk assessment. They used calcium and electron beam tomography because that was all that was available. The early work in coronary calcium scoring has led to a blinkered approach to risk assessment being validated predominantly through this method. There is complexity in bringing together a calcium score, a calcium score percentile, a description of the non-calcific plaque burden, including unfavourable positive remodelling, along with stenosis and the site of a lesion. This complexity is such that it has just not been able to have been broken down into a simple, reproducible, observational study or an interventional study. This was why I developed and use the C-PLUSS reporting approach but, due to its complexity and the variables involved, it is unlikely to ever be tested in a clinical trial.

General practitioners or family doctors are generally at the forefront of preventative care. Cardiac CT would fit well within their scope of care. Unfortunately, the technology has moved very quickly in recent years and this means few general practitioners have had exposure to its new developments. Also, as I discussed in the C-PLUSS chapter, unless the report to the family doctor is in a user-friendly language, then the significance of findings, particularly relating to future risk for the patient, may not be appreciated.

The patient's best interests are served by bringing together the expertise of all the above disciplines.

The radiologists have the most familiarity with CT technology and minimising radiation doses, while obtaining the best image quality.

The cardiologists have the most experience in understanding risk, dealing with the drugs involved in management and the best understanding of indications for revascularisation.

The patient's GP knows that patient and is in the best position to understand the personal circumstances of the individual, the family history, job stressors, exercise habits, social supports and other similar factors.

Pressures on the healthcare system

THIRDLY, cardiac CT imaging is not necessarily being used because of the pressures on our healthcare system.

	Urgent	Not Urgent
Important		
Not Important		

A matrix used originally by President Dwight Eisenhower is very useful in this discussion. Essentially, all activities can be placed into this simple matrix. There are things that are clearly **urgent** and these can fall into a category that is either **important** or **not important**. The **urgent-important** category would be dealing with someone having a heart attack. The **urgent-not-important** category might be a phone call – the phone ringing demands urgency although it may be a telemarketing call. Something that might fall in the **not-urgent-but-important** category could be putting in place the mechanisms required to reduce the risk of the population developing heart attacks. Something that might fit in the **not-urgent-not-important** category could be your intention to go through the last 30 years of Christmas photographs of your ex-in-laws and catalogue them.

The essence of this matrix is that most people (and organisations) spend most time in the urgent sectors. This means, importantly, we are often **not** in the **non-urgent-but-important** sector, the space required to put in place a cardiovascular disease prevention strategy.

....

I have already described that in the city I live we run a 24 hour a day, seven day per week angioplasty service to deal with acute coronary syndromes, or heart attacks. This is a fantastic service for a small city but has its price. There are only a handful of operators skilled in the procedure and so it is a finite resource. For the local public hospital to provide the service, it has to employ doctors who can do angioplasty so the load can be shared. For each position taken by an angioplasty cardiologist, there is one fewer space in the cardiology department for a cardiologist expert in another area, like prevention for example. I believe that because of the burden of MACE, pressures on public services are such that the acute care needs take priority. This is what you or I would want if we had a heart attack. It's just an unfortunate consequence of limited funds and resources. It leads to a situation akin to being busy, mopping up a flooded laundry without having the resources to turn off the tap that is causing the problem.

....

Business model

FOURTHLY, it's possible cardiac CT imaging is experiencing a slow take up because of **lack of familiarity and it threatens the current business model** used by cardiological services. This means that choices around selection of testing may be slightly skewed by the person recommending that test, based on that person's familiarity with, and financial interest in, the test.

I realised this early as the technology was being established in the local area through the radiology service. Initially I didn't support the service; I was unfamiliar with the technology and I derived no financial benefit from using it. Eventually I joined and worked with the radiology service to help expand the business. As I learnt more and became more familiar with the testing, I realised its value and started to use it more frequently. I could only do this if I could be sure there would be financial security in it for me, to reflect my investment of time and to reflect the lost income from other testing I could have been doing.

I make specific points when I speak with patients about cardiac CT imaging for risk assessment: that *firstly*, the testing is not covered by the Australian Government Health Insurance Commission and that *secondly,* I am paid to provide the reporting service for the testing. Without this personal business interest, I know that I would be unable to commit the time to learn and become familiar with the testing, less likely to refer to it and more likely to use stress testing, for example, for reassurance of patients, or even to progress to invasive coronary angiography to demonstrate the health of the arteries. While both these methods have been used for years, I believe they are sub-optimal compared with the potential prognostic value offered through cardiac CT imaging. I know from my own experience that cardiologists would not deliberately choose inappropriate tests for lack of comfort in a technology or for their own financial gain. However, I do wish to flag that having a financial interest in a particular technology, or not, may have an influence on the likelihood of developing familiarity with that test and referrals for that test at the time of clinical assessment.

Mindset

FIFTHLY, another challenge is **our mindset.** There is no question that humans deal with an emergency in a far more focussed way than we deal with planning to avoid an emergency. I know this from experience as a cardiologist. I have received lavish gratitude from patients who have presented in an acute, unstable setting and whose lives I have helped to save. This is dramatic, focussed, emotional and adrenaline-pumping. Good is being achieved.

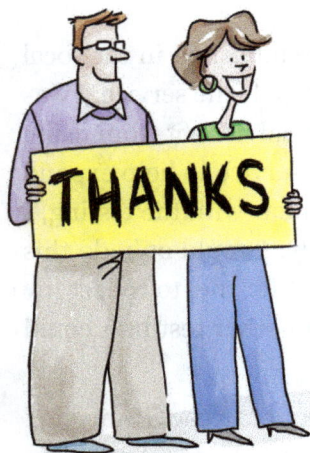

Throughout this book, however, I have written about preventative strategies and in this context I find the situation is quite different. An individual will come to me for an assessment or appraisal of his/her cardiovascular risk. The person will have no symptoms or problem at the time. Repeatedly, I have been in the situation when, over my office desk, in a controlled and organised way, I have explained that he or she carries an increased risk of an event. And because of this increased risk, he/she is likely to benefit from intervention with aspirin, cholesterol-lowering agents, perhaps blood pressure treatment and, in many cases lifestyle modification. I know that I am burdening this person with taking pills before anything has actually happened. I am sure that on many occasions patients have left my office wondering what it was all about, when they could have expressed gratitude that I may have averted a possible heart attack for them.

I would like to highlight that situation by a quote from a book, *The Black Swan,* by Nassim Nicholas Taleb.

A new kind of ingratitude

We remember the martyrs who died for a cause that we knew about, never those no less effective in their contribution but whose cause we were never aware of – precisely because they were successful. Our ingratitude toward the poètes maudits *fades completely in front of this other type of thanklessness. This is a far more vicious kind of ingratitude: the feeling of uselessness on the part of the silent hero. I will illustrate with the following thought experiment.*

Assume that a legislator with courage, influence, intellect, vision, and perseverance manages to enact a law that goes into universal effect and employment on September 10, 2001; it imposes the continuously locked bulletproof doors in every cockpit (at high costs to the struggling airlines) – just in case terrorists decide to use planes to attack the World Trade Center in

New York City. I know this is lunacy, but it is just a thought experiment (I am aware that there may be no such thing as a legislator with intellect, courage, vision, and perseverance; this is the point of the thought experiment). The legislation is not a popular measure among the airline personnel, as it complicates their lives. But it would certainly have prevented 9/11. The person who imposed locks on cockpit doors gets no statues in public squares, not so much as a quick mention of his contribution in his obituary. "Joe Smith, who helped avoid the disaster of 9/11, died of complications of liver disease." Seeing how superfluous his measure was, and how it squandered resources, the public, with great help from airline pilots, might well boot him out of office. Vox clamantis in deserto (meaning a voice crying out in the wilderness). He will retire depressed, with a great sense of failure. He will die with the impression of having done nothing useful. I wish I could go attend his funeral, but, reader, I can't find him. And yet, recognition can be quite a pump. Believe me, even those who genuinely claim that they do not believe in recognition, and that they separate labor from the fruits of labor, actually get a serotonin kick from it. See how the silent hero is rewarded: even his own hormonal system will conspire to offer no reward. Now consider again the events of 9/11. In their aftermath, who got the recognition? Those you saw in the media, on television performing heroic acts, and those whom you saw trying to give you the impression that they were performing heroic acts. The latter category includes someone like the New York Stock Exchange chairman Richard Grasso, who "saved the stock exchange" and received a huge bonus for his contribution (the equivalent of several thousand average salaries). All he had to do was be there to ring the opening bell on television – the television that, we will see, is the carrier of unfairness and a major cause of Black Swan blindness. Who gets rewarded, the central banker who avoids a recession or the one who comes to "correct" his predecessors' faults and happens to be there during some economic recovery? Who is more valuable, the politician who avoids a war or the one who starts a new one (and is lucky enough to win)? It is the same logic reversal we saw earlier with the value of what we don't know; everybody knows that you need more prevention than treatment, but few reward acts of prevention. We glorify those who left their names in history books at the expense of those contributors about whom our books are silent. We humans are not just a superficial race (this may be curable to some extent); we are a very unfair one.

This excerpt highlights beautifully the psyche and the emotion around our response to prevention and our response to disaster. It is just not sexy preventing heart attacks and I suggest cardiac CT suffers in this shadow!

Preconceived ideas from an earlier time

SIXTHLY, different pieces of information over time have filtered through and led to clinicians having **preconceived ideas** about the utility of cardiac CT imaging.

Radiation One of the main factors over the years has been a concern that the radiation dose is high. It was easy for someone who had not embraced the technology to simply say: "I believe the radiation dose is too high and I am unwilling to put my patients through that process." There was some truth in their concerns – initially. The earliest coronary angiograms used relatively high radiation doses, about 15 millisieverts, which is high but not off the scale in comparison with other medical imaging. A CT of the pelvis and chest, for example, carries a radiation exposure of between 5 and 10 millisieverts with a 1:2000 lifetime risk of developing a solid cell cancer[4].

The risk of cancer associated with radiation of 10mSv has been said to be 1:2000 lifetime risk of a solid cancer. This, however, is theoretical and extrapolated from higher doses received by atomic blast survivors. Studies on nuclear shipyard workers by British radiologists do not substantiate these statistical estimates[5]. Nonetheless, it is always best to err on the side of caution and keep radiation to a minimum (using the ALARA principle: As Low As Reasonably Achievable). In Australia workers exposed to radiation have limits of 20mSv per annum, averaged over five years, and an absolute limit of 50mSv in any one year[6].

To put this into context, there is radiation present in our daily lives all the time: rocky outcrops, electronic devices, atmospheric radiation, even radiation exposure while flying in a commercial aircraft. So, we are constantly being exposed to some degree of radiation. Background radiation, which is the term given to the radiation exposure of an individual human over a year through incidental exposure, is considered to run about three to five millisieverts per annum. So some degree of radiation exposure is normal in everyday life.

In the medical profession, the appropriate blanket approach is that we should absolutely minimise radiation exposure for an individual patient based on the particular clinical situation. Having said that, however, the lowest radiation dose for safety has not clearly been defined. In fact, there is even interesting data to suggest a small amount of extra radiation may not necessarily be a bad thing[7]. By way of comparison and reference, a mammogram, an x-ray of the breast tissue of a woman in a screening capacity undertaken on a regular basis almost, without second thought, carries with it a radiation exposure of approximately one millisievert. Flying in a commercial aircraft also carries with it exposure to radiation of approximately 0.1 millisieverts per hour in the air. For example, Sydney to London return is approximately 40 flying hours and so would expose a passenger to four millisieverts of radiation, about the same amount of radiation as a CT coronary angiogram.

Time, technology and medicine have moved on. Today, coronary calcium scoring can be undertaken with a radiation dose of one millisievert, akin to the same radiation exposure used in mammography as a screening test. It is not an unreasonable exposure when trying to bring clarity to management of the condition that still is responsible for 50 percent of all deaths in this country. As described earlier, if the calcium score is zero in the context of risk stratification, then further imaging may not be required. If the calcium score does show an abnormality and progression to coronary angiography is required, then most cardiac units in most centres with modern technology and modern techniques will be able to deliver a coronary angiogram with somewhere around four millisieverts or fewer. This is acceptable when we are dealing with a low lifetime risk of a possible solid tumour cancer versus the importance of knowing the status of someone's coronary arteries in the context of having demonstrated calcification. For the Western world's greatest killer, an awareness of the radiation dose is important but has to be seen in balance.

Negative publicity   In Australia, some practitioners adopted the technology before the technology was ready to be adopted. Around 1998, an enthusiastic early adopter began scanning people's hearts using a two slice CT scanner, on the back of the work being done by the likes of Agatston using electron beam tomography. The intent was good in that he clearly understood that if calcium could be identified on electron beam tomography to help in risk stratification, then using an alternate type of CT scanner to demonstrate calcification would certainly offer potentially useful information. However, suggesting that a two slice CT scanner could perform the same job as an electron beam scanner was like suggesting a Volkswagen Beetle could perform just as well as an F1 Mercedes: different machines, different leagues. Although he found patients who had calcium in their arteries and was able to implement follow-on strategies, he raised the ire of the local medical community. One concern was that he was using a multi-slice scanner when all the evidence had been collected for electron beam tomography. A fair comment: VW vs F1. It was also noted that as people get older, calcium becomes more prevalent and at that stage there were no nomograms (tables) to guide percentiles for individuals, based on specific age or sex. The other concern raised by the medical fraternity was the issue of knock-on testing which was seen potentially to be a money-making exercise. I am sure, though, that the doctor would have had many anecdotal cases in which that knock-on testing led to intervention and a positive benefit for the patient.

The situation was such that it led to an eminent representative of the Cardiac Society of Australia and New Zealand (CSANZ) discussing the situation through public media, including the ABC health report. Public representation by this generally conservative body is almost unprecedented. He also wrote an article published in the *New England Journal of Medicine* (a very highly regarded medical journal) at the end of 1999, which flagged that calcification alone was not necessarily well correlated with stenosis, that more information was needed for event rates and more information was needed for intervention. That negative exposure over 15 years ago in the local press (in which the medical fraternity, in an organised and structured way, quite reasonably raised concerns about a particular intervention and the way it was being used) has left a cloud in the psyche of medical practitioners who were exposed to the coverage, to this day. This means that current evaluation of the technology is viewed through a prism of suspicion and mistrust.

Since that time, however, the situation has changed dramatically. Data now exist that correlate multi-detector CT scanning with electron beam tomography, such that on the current modern 64 (or more) slice scanners the acquisition of a coronary calcium score is completely and utterly validated, based on the original works. Significant amounts of data have been collected to allow an understanding of calcium score related to age and sex and there are comprehensive charts available to provide calcium score percentiles for individual patients. Increasingly more robust data supporting event rates, particularly around the use of coronary calcium scoring alone, are available.

Overall, many of the concerns raised, quite appropriately in 1999, have faded with time and the acquisition of further data around the technology and improvements in the technology. The impact of the negative publicity, however, does not appear to have faded to the same extent.

IMPORTANT POINTS

- There are hurdles that obstruct broad use of cardiac CT:
  » Supporting studies may never be done.
  » Radiologists, cardiologists and local doctors see the technology differently.
  » Its implementation is 'not urgent but important', meaning that it does not receive priority.
  » A change in familiarity and in the business model would be needed for some practitioners.
  » Do we respond to a crisis or do we prevent a crisis?
  » Early issues with radiation dose and bad publicity linger in the minds of many medical practitioners who could be using the technology.

[1]   Arad Y, Spadaro LA, Roth M, Newstein D, Guerci AD. Treatment of asymptomatic
        adults with elevated coronary calcium scores with atorvastatin, vitamin C, and
        vitamin E: the St. Francis Heart Study randomized clinical trial. J Am Coll Cardiol
        2005;46:166-72.

[2]   Arbab-Zadeh A, Miller JM, Rochitte CE, et al. Diagnostic Accuracy of Computed
        Tomography Coronary Angiography According to Pre-Test Probability of Coronary
        Artery Disease and Severity of Coronary Arterial CalcificationThe CORE-64 (Coronary
        Artery Evaluation Using 64-Row Multidetector Computed Tomography Angiography)
        International Multicenter Study. J Am Coll Cardiol 2012;59:379-87.

[3]   Meijboom WB, Meijs MFL, Schuijf JD, et al. Diagnostic Accuracy of 64-Slice Computed
        Tomography Coronary Angiography A Prospective, Multicenter, Multivendor Study.
        J Am Coll Cardiol 2008;52:2135-44.

[4]   Frenz MB, Mee AS. Diagnostic radiation exposure and cancer risk. Gut 2005;
        54:889-90.

[5]   Berrington A, Darby S, Weiss H, Doll R. 100 years of observation on British
        radiologists: mortality from cancer and other causes 1897–1997. The British Journal
        of Radiology 2001;74:507-19.

[6]   Boice Jr JD, Cohen SS, Mumma MT, et al. Updated mortality analysis of radiation
        workers at Rocketdyne (Atomics International), 1948-2008. Radiation research
        2011;176:244-58.

[7]   Chen W, Luan Y, Shieh M, et al. Is chronic radiation an effective prophylaxis against
        cancer? Journal of American Physicians and Surgeons 2004;9:6.

pages 194-5 credit: The Black Swan: The Impact of the Highly Improbable by
Nassim Nicholas Taleb (Penguin Books, 2008) Copyright © Nassim Nicholas Taleb, 2007

Even good ideas come at a price. The next chapter looks at the hard reality of money. Is primary preventive medicine, as outlined in this book, worth the cash needed to support it?

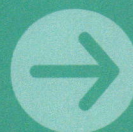

→

Chapter 17 -
At what cost?

IN THIS CHAPTER WE LOOK AT

> the cost of screening:

- can we afford it?

- can we afford not to screen?

I have suggested that there is scope to use cardiac CT imaging as a screening tool for risk stratification, to improve cardiovascular risk management. We have discussed the lack of randomised controlled trials and the presence of observational studies as the evidence base to guide risk assessment and management. Concerns regarding radiation dose and contrast dose are constantly being addressed and re-evaluated, with improved technology reducing radiation dose. More recently, new protocols looking at reducing contrast load have also come into play[1].

So, if we consider cardiac CT imaging as a way forward, we also have to consider the cost, not just to the individual but to the community. Although my expertise is not in health economics, I offer the following figures as a starting point for consideration and further discussion.

So, let's consider again our one hundred 50-year-old men. Of these 100 men with intermediate risk (15 percent risk of MACE in 10 years), 15 will have an event and 85 will not. If we use imaging to find the 15 who have the worst arteries and the 85 who are not so bad, we can then consider the most appropriate way to manage the 100 and so work out some costs.

Cost of screening and treatment

CALCIUM SCORE We know from previous discussions around coronary calcium score that 25 percent of men at 50 years of age will have a zero calcium score. If we screen our 100 patients and find the 25 with a zero calcium score, no further evaluation will be required, as all the research data suggest that this group carries a low risk of event over the next 10 years.

COST If we were to use a figure of $300 per coronary calcium score, then 100 patients would cost $30,000 (100 x $300).

CCTA This leaves 75 patients to be evaluated with a CCTA, knowing that within that 75 there are at least 15 who will be high to very high risk.

COST If we use a cost of $700 for the CCTA, then the cost to screen the remaining 75 individuals is $52,500 (75 x $700).

This combination, of calcium scoring and CCTA, will yield a range of results. So now we have:-

- used calcium scoring and/or coronary angiography on 100 patients;
- yielded 25 with a zero score – no further action required;
- undertaken 75 full cardiac CTs, and
- defined:
  » 15 highest calcium scores, the group most likely to have a heart attack in the next 10 years;
  » 10 who sit between the 75th and 85th percentile who run an increased risk of heart attack, particularly over the next 10 to 15 years;
  » 5 to 10 who have features on their cardiac scan which are substantially higher risk than suggested by their calcium score alone (a subset who could have a MACE contrary to their calcium score alone), and
  » about 40 to 45 with 'in-between' findings.

At this stage, CCS + CCTA, we have incurred a total cost of $82,500 ($30,000 plus $52,500) to define what I believe is the most accurate cardiovascular risk stratification for those individuals over the following 10 years.

Some of the men, however, will require further appropriate management at additional cost:

- The 15 who are high- to very high-risk should receive statin therapy. Statins, the main class of cholesterol-lowering drugs, have come off patent and generic brands are now cheaply available in Australia so that therapy can be achieved for as little as $16 per month. The cost per annum would be $16/month x 12 months x 10 years x the 15 patients: $31,000-32,000 for the high- to very high-risk individuals. As these figures are only a rough estimate and aspirin is cheap, I have included aspirin in these costs.

- The lowest risk 25 do not need drugs.

- However, if we were to also treat patients who fall above the 75th percentile for calcium scores, because they are in the highest quarter for age and sex, then it is likely that an extra 10 patients would warrant therapy. The cost of this would be $16/month x 12 months x 10 years x 10 patients, or close to $20,000.

- Further to that, there will be perhaps up to 5 to 10 percent of patients whose risk from CCTA is far greater than that envisaged from coronary calcium scoring alone. Say there were seven patients to be treated, at $16/month each x 12 months x 10 years, including aspirin, the cost would be $13,000-$14,000.

Bringing all those costs together – for the scanning of 100 patients using coronary calcium scoring as a gatekeeper, such that 75 go on to CCTA for further risk stratification and then, having risk-stratified, selecting 30 patients out of that 100 to treat – **the cost of scans and of treatment is in the order of $150,000 over that 10 year period.**

Remember from the last chapter, this incurred the risk of a very small chance of developing a solid tumour during a lifetime and a risk of 1:100,000 of a life-ending allergic (anaphylactic) reaction. Coronary artery disease still accounts for approximately 50 percent of all deaths in the Western world.

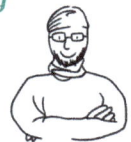

Cost of a heart attack

If we come back to our initial 100 patients who are 50 years of age with intermediate risk, and understand that approximately 15 events will occur in that 100, and within those 15 events, we estimate conservatively that there will be one death and that there will be one major heart attack with significant damage to the heart muscle such that the individual is rendered significantly affected for the rest of his life, then we can start to put the costs of screening and treatment into context with the costs borne by the individuals and the community.

We have just spent close to $150,000 hopefully to prevent 15 MACE, including the unexpected death of one man aged between 50 and 60 years of age. Even if we accept we can't prevent all events, and conservatively estimate preventing 30 percent of events, is this expensive? I am not in a position to put a price on one death but to loved ones and the community it is significant.

For the one individual who has the heart attack with significant damage to his heart, the costs are easier to determine: an ambulance (several hundred dollars), A&E presentation (hundreds of dollars), potentially urgent transfer out-of-hours to a coronary invasive angiography unit for acute stenting (thousands of dollars including cost of stent, staff and theatre on call, and disposables), then the cost of the hospital ($500-600 per night). It is easy to see thousands, and even tens of thousands, of dollars mounting up very quickly. Let's say the overall cost is $10,000 for the acute admission to hospital with a heart attack – and this does not include the loss of work or impact on lifestyle for the individual patient. If there is damage to the heart then there may be a need for complicated therapies which include drug therapies and also implantable devices (special defibrillators to reduce the risk of sudden death due to electrical malfunction of the heart in the future) and multiple visits to outpatient clinics for management of medical issues, as well as ongoing management of the implanted devices. When some of these implanted devices alone can cost between $30,000 and $50,000, it is easy to see that one patient with a complicated course of treatment can lead to significant costs being borne by the community.

Importantly, in this approach, cholesterol medication is not being prescribed for patients who don't need it. These are patients who may have high cholesterol but no predisposition to a build-up of atheroma in the arteries. This is a saving that can be fed back into the system.

It is also important to be aware of the cost the community currently pays for different aspects of health care. Haemodialysis (kidney dialysis) is generally considered the yardstick of acceptable expenditure for one life. This currently runs at close to $90,000 per annum. When seen in comparison, screening the initial 100 men doesn't seem that expensive, does it?

Although not based on a thorough economic evaluation, my feeling is that the costs of scanning and treatment in this group of one hundred 50-year-old men with a 15 percent risk of event over 10 years is a very good deal. It reduces personal hardship but also has the potential to significantly avert costly medical interventions.

In time, no doubt, more thorough cost evaluations will be made as a guide for communities and countries in developing their health policies. In the interim, the decision really rests with the individual patient to decide whether or not the investigation is personally cost effective.

IMPORTANT POINTS

- What value would you put on saving one life?
- What value would you put on preventing one debilitating event?
- Do you think prevention is cheaper than cure?

[1] Oda S, Utsunomiya D, Yuki H, et al. Low contrast and radiation dose coronary CT angiography using a 320-row system and a refined contrast injection and timing method. J Cardiovasc Comput Tomogr 2015;9:19-27.

The next chapter explains why the news is always GOOD news.

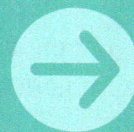

Testimonial

I was very pleased to have been referred to Dr Warrick Bishop.

I'd always had slightly high cholesterol levels but when I hit 60, my heart risk rating jumped up and my doctor wanted to put me on statins. I asked if there was any other choice to this, as I wasn't keen on life-long medication. She referred me to Dr Bishop who explained that he had a way to make a more educated assessment of whether I was one of the 20 per cent of people in my risk profile who could benefit from statins, or not.

To this end I went through the cardiac CT scan procedure which showed an anomaly of plaque build-up and narrowing in one of my arteries. Warrick was concerned enough to put me through a second round of testing involving a treadmill for an exercise stress echocardiogram, involving an ultrasound designed to show if there was any restriction of blood flow through that particular artery. To my relief, the test proved negative. The plaque is there but it's not constricting blood flow.

All this has shown that it is important for me to take statins and aspirin- and importantly, be on an improved low-carbohydrate food regime.

So, in the end, I wasn't able to avoid the on-going medication. Of course, I might have gone on to the medication straight away via my own doctor, avoiding the cardiac tests. However, I then would not have been any wiser as to the condition in that pesky artery and the serious risk that it presents. Now I know what is going on, I am the wiser for it.

I am very pleased with the final outcome; that has been very reassuring. I found Warrick Bishop to be very attentive, always explaining things clearly, patiently and in simple terms. The tests were straightforward and not too time consuming; the staff at the Calvary Hospital in Hobart are all wonderfully friendly and caring.

If you have any concerns about your heart health, then I strongly recommend that you see Dr Warrick Bishop.

Paul Archer

Chapter 18 -
Planning your own heart attack (NOT!)

IN THIS CHAPTER WE LOOK AT

> making your own plans:
- do you want to be forewarned and prepared?
> what's the alternative?

By now you will have learnt a little bit about the heart and the coronary arteries. You now know about atherosclerotic plaque, how it can be calcific dominant or 'cholesterol' or non-calcific dominant, and how its build-up can be patchy through the arteries.

You understand that traditional risk factors are important but still don't tell you what is going on in **your** arteries. Eating a 'healthy diet', exercising, not being overweight are all good things but they do not necessarily protect you. They only help predict risk in a population of individuals with the same characteristics.

You also realise that elevated cholesterol isn't always associated with problems in the arteries. You may be in the position of wanting to know if a statin that has been recommended for you is really required based on what is going on in **your** arteries.

You are aware of the reassurance of a zero coronary calcium score (for men over 50 and women over 60 years of age) and how, if there is calcium present in the arteries, undertaking CCTA will provide the most accurate way to assess plaque specific characteristics. You know that combining the calcium score with the calcium score percentile, then looking at plaque specific characteristics will provide the most information to make a risk assessment from the cardiac CT scan. This needs to be integrated with the individual's clinical characteristics. Treatment is then based on the combination of the patient's traditional risk features and the plaque-specific risk features.

I have employed this approach with 2500-3000 patients over the past five years. To date, I have not had a single out-of-hospital cardiac arrest in the patients who have remained on the prescribed medication and continued with appropriate follow up.

....

You have some choice in this. The more informed you are, the better the choices you can make.

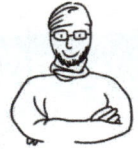

....

The 2013 ACC/AHA (American College of Cardiology/American Heart Association) guideline on the assessment of cardiovascular risk covers the topic of traditional risk factors comprehensively. That recommendation says that adults between 20 and 79 years of age should be evaluated every four years using traditional risk factors. If their 10 year risk is greater than 7.5 percent then they should be evaluated into a high-risk category; if their risk is less than 7.5 percent, then a 30 year lifetime risk can be evaluated[1].

In Australia, we use the Australian Cardiovascular Risk Disease Calculator which includes age, sex, total cholesterol level, HDL cholesterol, smoking status, diabetes status and presence of left ventricular hypertrophy (which is thickening of the heart muscle) on ECG. *(http://www.cvdcheck.org.au/)* Interestingly, neither the American nor Australian traditional risk factor calculators include family history, diet, exercise, weight nor waist-to-hip ratio. Both American and Australian approaches are based on populations and both have the inherent limitations of that approach. **They are excellent for predicting within a population but not for the individual.**

The thrust of this book is to raise awareness around the possibility of using cardiac CT imaging as a way to look at a population and find the *individuals* within that population who would be at higher or lower risk than the average of that population.

My approach is to routinely scan men at 50 years of age and women at 60 years of age, as it tends to be the following 10 to 15 years when the majority of unexpected cardiac events occur in the intermediate-risk population. My observation is that there tends to be family clusters and so I lower the 50/60 age if there is a significant family history of premature coronary artery disease, particularly if associated with unfavourable risk markers. I consider scanning the individual patient 5 to 10 years earlier than the family's first event to ensure we are ahead of the game. The other situation in which I consider earlier scanning for risk is if there are significant traditional risks (for example, very high cholesterol, obesity, pre-diabetes, diabetes, high blood pressure, being a smoker) that could mean a young patient may be carrying a significant likelihood of a heart attack. The timing of this, I believe, is a specialist area and would warrant the patient seeing a cardiologist with an interest in cardiac CT imaging and prevention. This would ensure the most appropriate use of the technology and the best possible interpretation of the results.

In general, I tend to be more interested in the lipid profile (cholesterol levels and different lipoprotein levels) **after** the scan results, as this shows what is going on in the arteries and is our guide to intervention. Lipid issues should be discussed with someone who has interest and knowledge in the field.

Before undertaking any screening, it is important for a patient to be aware that knock-on effects may result from the scan. I make a point of explaining to patients that because insurance companies do not have a clear understanding of where this technology fits, an abnormality could have a detrimental impact on a person's ability to obtain re-insurance. To that end, I recommend that patients who are about to undergo cardiac CT imaging for risk stratification speak with their insurance brokers to obtain information around what impact the findings of the scan may have on their insurance. Not only does this forewarn them but it also allows them to put appropriate guaranteed, renewable insurance in place, if necessary. I do not try to cover the detail of insurance with patients, as it is not my area of expertise, but I do feel an obligation to raise it as an issue that needs to be considered before obtaining information which would need to be considered as part of a full disclosure.

Similarly, there are some occupations in which interpretation of findings related to atheroma build-up on cardiac CT scan could have an untoward effect on accreditation, certification or licensing. For example, the finding of a significant atheroma burden in a commercial pilot could well lead to a request for further testing or evaluation by the licensing board. To be aware of these issues prior to undertaking the initial investigation is nothing more than being prepared.

However, one should not lose sight of the main objective here. Not checking your heart because of possible problems with insurance or licensing could result in your paperwork being in order but you are no longer here!

Lastly, in relation to the evaluation of chest pain (particularly sudden onset [A&E-type] chest pain which arises as a symptom occurring *de novo*), my strong recommendation is to explore whether the particular situation is one that could be evaluated using cardiac CT imaging, so that not only a diagnosis of anatomical significance is provided *(Is there a narrowing or not?)* but also information that would yield prognostic information *(Is there a significant atheroma burden that could mean increased risk of a heart attack in the future?).*

Whatever the news, it's good news

I have had patients and even colleagues say to me they just don't want to know what's going on with their heart. They don't want to know in case it is bad news. Well, I can understand this as a knee-jerk response but really it is ostrich behaviour. Sticking your head in the sand is not going to solve anything, nor allow sensible planning, whatever the situation may be. I say to these 'ostriches', "Do you have your car serviced? If you do, why?" The choice between finding out about brakes that may fail during a scheduled service

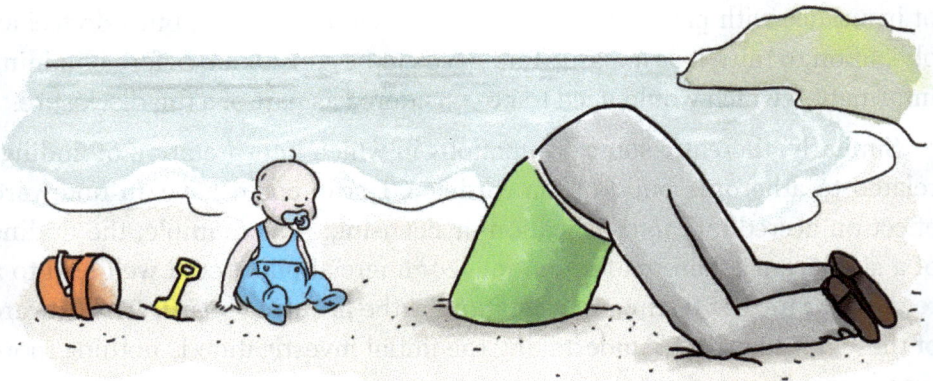

or on a drive during a family holiday is a no-brainer. The chance to find out about potential problems can provide confronting information but what's the alternative?

There are only fours ways to diagnose coronary artery plaque:

1) At the time of autopsy. *Too late.*

2) In the back of an ambulance on the way to hospital. *Still too late.*

3) With chest pain and shortness of breath. *Late in the process.*

4) Cardiac CT imaging – **before a problem has occurred.**

How would you want to find out?

Doctors have told me that they have had patients with high-risk findings on their scan who then suffer because of anxiety created by the findings. In my experience, this is very uncommon. I make a particular point of explaining to patients about to undergo the scan that "whatever the result, it will be helpful information". My experience is that a clear discussion with education and expectations prior to and support after the test means the results of the scan are dealt with objectively, expending minimal emotional energy. Some patients will have an anxiety disorder which needs treatment anyway and, if it weren't the scan result, it would be something else causing concern. And sure, some doctors could learn to improve their delivery. Either way, this should not detract from the big picture.

If the scan shows low-risk features – great!

Off you go.

If the scan shows high-risk features – great!

This is what we are going to do to reduce that risk...

Ultimately, individuals will deal with situations differently and sometimes there is little that can be done to change that. My feeling and experience, however, is that for the vast majority of patients, dealing with the facts in a sensible, balanced way makes for good sense and good medicine.

Plan your heart attack (NOT!)

- **I recommend screening:** at 50 years of age for men unless there is a significant risk factor at play and, for women, as they tend to follow men's risk by about 10 years, at 60, again unless other risk factors come into play.

- You will need to **discuss screening with your regular doctor.** The doctor may not be familiar enough with the technology to answer all your questions, or may not be comfortable with requesting the test through lack of experience with it. You may need to see a cardiologist with an interest in the area, someone like me, who can best assess your needs and make the appropriate arrangements for heart rate control which is required for optimal scanning. I see many patients in this capacity.

- You will need to find a centre that has the **right equipment**: a minimum of a 64 slice CT scanner. Your referring doctor should know this.

- It is best to have a centre that has **both a radiologist and a cardiologist** onsite, as both bring different skills to acquiring the test and its quality.

- That centre also needs to have **experience** obtaining the images with **good image quality** and **low radiation doses.** Have your scan done at a high-volume centre that concentrates on best image quality at lowest achievable radiation doses. Again, your referring doctor should know this.

- Once you have had the scan, then it needs to be **reported** in a way that relates to the risk features demonstrated. I recommend the C-PLUSS approach in addition to the report fulfilling the SCCT guidelines.

- The results of the scan then need to be discussed with you and a **plan for future management** made. Some local doctors may have the experience to deal with this, particularly if the findings are straightforward; some won't. I see it as a very important part of the care I provide for a patient through the screening process.

- If your results are high- to very high-risk, **see a cardiologist.**

Remember, whatever the result, it's GREAT.

IMPORTANT POINTS ✔

- For the reader who is the patient ...

  » You have a choice in your care and the ongoing management of your situation.

  » Gather as much information as possible.

  » Understand the risk and benefits **for you!**

  » Deal with doctors or specialists with cardiac CT experience.

  » I wish you all the best!

[1] *Eckel RH, Jakicic JM, Ard JD, et al. 2013 AHA/ACC Guideline on Lifestyle Management to Reduce Cardiovascular Risk: A Report of the American College of Cardiology/American Heart Association Task Force on Practice Guidelines. Circulation 2014;129:S76-S99.*

The next chapter encourages you to join the conversation and be part of changing medical practice.

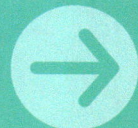

Testimonial

I am 52 years of age, work in an office position and have always struggled with my weight. That, combined with a family history of heart disease, has worried me that I could die prematurely of a heart-related condition. In recent years I have managed to drop my weight by about 28kg (adopting a low carbohydrate eating plan for some of this weight loss) and have incorporated exercise into my daily routine. However, I always had in the back of my mind that I still could have a high risk of suffering a heart attack.

I visited my GP in January 2015 for a general check-up and discussed the cardiac CT scanning idea with her. My GP ran the online cardiovascular disease risk calculator which resulted in my having a one percent risk of heart attack but, because of the family history, we discussed that cardiac CT scanning would be a positive thing for me to do. I had read about it before and had always managed to find an excuse not to go through with it; this year something made me decide that I had to do it.

I made the appointment with Dr Bishop and went along for my routine blood tests beforehand. I had thought for a while that I probably should have been taking medication to lower my cholesterol although, when I had been to another GP two years previously, I was told that because I had no other symptoms, it was probably not necessary. After I received my blood test results my cholesterol, which has see-sawed over the last few years, had gone up to 6.1, so I knew that I needed to finally do something about it.

My husband came along with me to my first appointment to see Warrick Bishop and, by the end of the consultation, we had both decided to undergo the cardiac CT testing. We agreed with Dr Bishop that it would be a win-win situation to find out our risk factors and go on to medication if necessary.

I was hoping for a miracle; I hoped that I had been worrying for nothing. My husband was sceptical that it was going to be worth it.

A couple of weeks after our scans, at our follow-up appointment with Dr Bishop, my worst fears were realised. Dr Bishop explained what he had seen from my results: I had a substantial build-up of cholesterol in my arteries and my risk of heart attack was extremely high. If left untreated, I stood a high chance of having an "episode" as he put it within five years. I needed to go on to a very strong dose of cholesterol-lowering medication immediately, and he wanted to follow up with me within three months to see if the medication was making a difference. Needless to say it was a big wake-up call for me. My husband, on the other hand, had great results: no build up in his arteries and no need for medication at that time.

I have been on medication to lower my cholesterol now for three months, and after having another series of more investigative blood tests, at my latest visit Dr Bishop told me my cholesterol has dropped to 4.1. Dr Bishop is happy with my results and does not want to see me for 12 months.

I will need to continue with my medication for the rest of my life but considering what could have happened if I had continued blindly along the road on which I was headed, it may be have been a very different story.

To say that cardiac CT scanning has been a life saving experience for me is an understatement. If I had continued to put my head in the sand and not had the scan, who knows what may have happened. I am not out of the woods but am now more aware that, should I experience any symptoms of heart attack, I need to act on them quickly. It could be the difference between life and death.

I am extremely glad and very fortunate that this testing was available for my husband and me, and I extend my thanks to Dr Bishop for his encouragement and belief in this procedure.

Caroline Harding

What has this all been for?
Prevention is better than cure.

'Prevention is better than cure' and Dr Warrick Bishop's book illustrates how our patients can prevent a heart attack. This comprehensive book will not only serve as a wake-up call for many people, but also save lives.

Dr Bishop has managed to make a complicated subject easy to understand for everyone, with descriptive examples and illustrations. I will certainly be recommending this book to my patients.

Karam Kostner

Associate Professor of Medicine, University of Queensland

and Director of Cardiology, Mater Hospital

Brisbane, Queensland, Australia

Dr Karam Kostner's clinical interest is preventative cardiology and lipid disorders. He has also been actively involved in cardiovascular research for 15 years, mainly in the area of lipoproteins, lipid lowering and atherosclerosis.

Having published approximately 90 peer reviewed papers, four book chapters and several review articles and editorials, Dr Kostner has also given numerous invited lectures at cardiovascular meetings. He is secretary of the Cardiac Society of Australia and NZ, Queensland branch, having also been president. He is an editorial board member and section editor of the European Journal of Clinical Investigation, and a regular reviewer for many journals, as well as being a NHMRC Grant Reviewer. Dr Koster has also organised or been on the committee of several national and international conferences.

Chapter 19 -
The future

> beginning a conversation that will encourage:

- the widespread use of cardiac CT imaging so that it will be included in public health policy

- ongoing research into understanding, treatment and management of coronary artery disease

- government and regulatory bodies to reconsider their approach to proactive lessening of risk

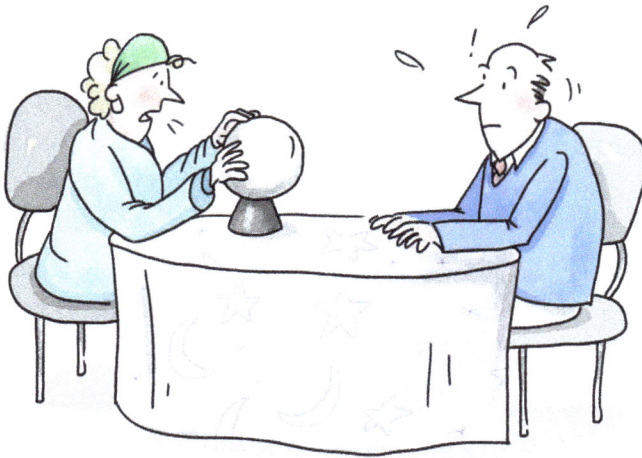

"It's telling me that a cardiac CT will do a better job of predicting your future!"

My hope from this book is to begin a conversation which ultimately increases utilisation of cardiac CT imaging, in combination with other risk factor evaluation, in order to improve primary prevention for coronary artery disease.

My vision is that imaging will be incorporated into a more holistic approach, thus improving the way we deal with the potential risk many individuals carry in regard to coronary artery disease. As this technology becomes more familiar to the community, then its use could be at the coalface for general practitioners who are, by virtue of their position in providing medical care, the custodians of preventative medicine.

Cardiac CT imaging could become the preferred tool of risk assessment for general practitioners in a way that allows the technology to appropriately guide intervention or allows a choice regarding a modified approach in an individual patient. However, until clear-cut guidelines are established, it may be that specialist involvement will be important for the most appropriate use of the technology.

As we are comfortable with mammography for breast screening, pap smears for population screening, measuring cholesterol levels and blood sugar levels, my hope is that we will see cardiac CT imaging as one of the tools available for widespread implementation in public policy.

My hope also is that there is recognition of imaging findings to help guide government-supported statin prescription, which currently in Australia is based on traditional criteria alone. This excludes a group of patients with lower intermediate-risk factor profile but high-risk features on cardiac CT imaging. It makes sense to focus treatment on what is going on in the arteries of an individual patient, not what **may** be going on in the arteries based on probability.

There will be issues regarding cost, efficacy and appropriateness. Of course, there will be studies in the future that will answer some of these questions, while for others, the study may never be done.

Widespread public screening presents the opportunity to evaluate the state of an individual person's arteries and make appropriate decisions, which are particular and specific for that individual. My feeling is it should not rely on the population in which the person sits statistically to decide the care; cardiac CT imaging allows us to be more precise than that.

The future may look at repeat scanning as an appropriate tool to assess intervention. Although the current data is not clear cut, there is some research to support it[1]. In my practice, there are specific situations in which I think it is appropriate and, at this stage, it is a management strategy that is best left to specialist interpretation.

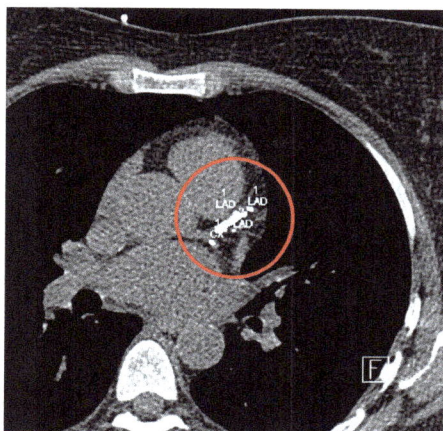

An individual who has 'a lot' of calcium in the arteries in both absolute terms, and in age and sex terms.

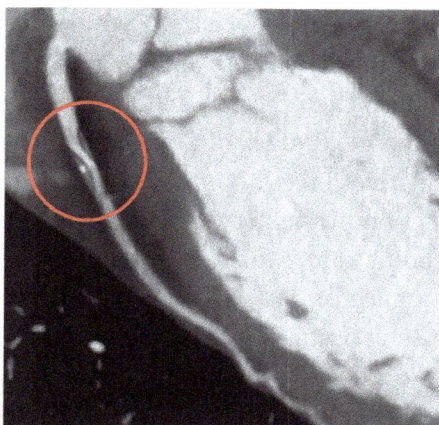

An example in which there is little calcium but considerable non-calcific (cholesterol-rich) plaque. A single plaque in the proximal LAD that leads to a MACE is 'affectionately' known as a 'widow maker'.

As the use of imaging the coronary arteries increases, there is no doubt in my mind that improved understanding of the underlying process of coronary atheroma will develop. In the simplest of terms, we see situations when there is a significant widespread presence of atheroma in the arteries and this is manifest with a significant calcium burden, reflective of the process of atheroma accumulation within the arteries. At the same time, however, imaging clearly demonstrates situations when minimal calcium is deposited within the arteries in the setting of significant build-up of cholesterol.

The more we image these two different ends of the spectrum and the more data we collect around these situations, the better will be our understanding and, therefore, our management into the future. We may start to be able to predict an individual's propensity to form one type of plaque or the other. One day we may even be able to predict at what location in the artery plaque is likely to occur. Wouldn't that be amazing? Only time and continued observation will facilitate this process.

Cardiac CT imaging also demonstrates situations when only one plaque exists within the entire coronary circulation. However, the location of that plaque (for example in the proximal part of the left anterior descending artery, also known as a 'widow maker') is such that rupture of that plaque can be catastrophic. I have searched the literature and spoken with experts from all over the world for an explanation of this process. I have not been able to find a good explanation, and certainly no way to predict its presence – without imaging.

My feeling is that it is probably related to local shear stress within the artery as a consequence of the path the LAD takes over the fibrous ring that separates the top part of the heart (atria) from the bottom part of the heart (ventricles). With each contraction of the heart, there is a point above the fibrous ring where the artery remains relatively fixed compared with the artery running over the ventricle. The junction of the moving and relatively fixed parts of the LAD creates a hinge point that can be subject to local stress, causing wear and tear. The consequence of this wear and tear is the development of a localised plaque. This doesn't occur in everyone thankfully, and is probably related to specific features of the path which the LAD takes. This might be a little like a scenario in which some people with knock knees develop arthritis. Some people with bow knees get arthritis. Yet most people with straight legs probably won't have arthritis of their knees. With time and greater understanding, we may be advocating treatment of a single plaque well before an event occurs. (There is some research looking into this.)

Localised plaque is challenging. There are occasions when I have recommended that a patient take statin and aspirin for a single high-risk plaque. The plaque may be no more than 15mm in length, so the patient is going to be taking 'lifelong' treatment for one small but significant spot of cholesterol build-up. It almost seems out of proportion that a person will take a medication that will inevitably find its way through every organ of his body in order to address a single small patch of atheroma. Unfortunately, this is the best we have at the moment.

BUT … What if, in the future, we developed antibodies which are specific to the mechanisms behind plaque development? Could we inject a serum of antibodies that would arrest the progression of plaque formation *in situ?* If it worked for a single plaque, could it work for more extensive disease? What if we could develop nano technology that could target the plaque and remove the debris and cholesterol, leaving a safe but tiny scar in the artery? What a thought: a simple injection or course of injections, to arrest the process that currently rates as the leading cause of death in Western countries! Or, it may be that we observe and understand that early stenting of a high risk, single plaque positively affects the outcome. Whichever way medical technology develops, although coronary artery disease is the single most studied human condition, we are at the beginning of those processes of observation and understanding and will have to wait until the future unveils more clarity.

Moving on

Let's not get ahead of ourselves, as exciting as the prospect might be. There are issues that can and should be addressed now. The experience of our friend, Bill, from earlier in the book, represents an excellent example of how our current approach to atheroma burden and its management requires realignment. This realignment is not only within the medical area but also within the greater community and, for this particular case, specifically within the insurance industry.

Bill's plight is representative of a very significant point: that knowing the health of one's arteries and acting accordingly is far better than having no idea and responding to disaster. **The sooner insurance companies can get their heads around this and *not* penalise patients who proactively seek to maximise their future cardiac risk management, the better.** I would suggest that the same companies would do well to realise that the stress tests they have relied on for years are no longer the best tool available for defining risk. It is time to move with the changes in technology and the benefit of improved risk modelling, so that cheaper premiums, but most importantly better health outcomes, are available for everyone.

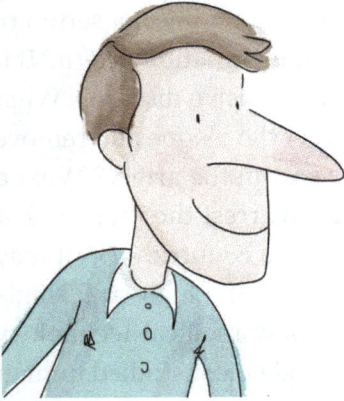

So, remember Bill, who, in the context of a borderline family history of MACE, requested cardiac CT imaging at the age of 48. Scanning was undertaken and it demonstrated a surprisingly high coronary calcium score, in fact, above the 90th percentile for age and sex. CCTA demonstrated high- to very high-risk features with possible flow limitation of the circumflex artery. His stress test at the time was negative for flow limitation. Bill, after also undergoing screening bloods for high-risk factors, ended up taking aspirin, statin, nicotinic acid (he had a low HDL cholesterol and a high lipoprotein a), ACE inhibitor, vitamin D and fish oil. He undertakes very regular exercise; his exercise capacity is such that he has trained for and completed the equivalent of an Hawaiian Ironman event. He also keeps an eye on a reduced carbohydrate eating guideline. As he did not tolerate statin well, he was on a very low dose every second or third day.

In the setting of full disclosure, Bill notified his insurance company of the findings of his cardiac CT scan. This lead to his insurance company not re-negotiating his policies. He was 'pinned down' by being proactive and looking after himself. It resulted in more restrictions and more focus on his lipid profile, which interestingly had never been that much of a problem. This response could only be described as disappointing.

The reality is that his risk, post-scan, had been more than halved with education and preventative strategies, yet his insurance company responded rigidly. It refused any re-negotiation of his policy. This is not only the wrong way around but sends the wrong message to an individual who may want to be proactive in the care of his cardiovascular health. Luckily, Bill didn't think twice about what his scan may show and what his insurer may do. He realised the information, whatever it was going to be, would benefit him and his family and that there was no point keeping his insurance premiums unchanged at the risk of dropping dead prematurely.

In Bill's situation, the context of not being able to treat as we had hoped, nor achieve the desired lower lipid levels[2], we undertook stress testing as a potential indicator of progression that could lead to narrowing (this is not stress testing to define risk). Several years into Bill's on-going management plan, with on-going surveillance stress testing, we clearly demonstrated a problem. Within the week, Bill had undergone invasive coronary angiography and had a stent inserted into the proximal circumflex artery which resulted in a full re-establishment of blood flow to that area of the myocardium, with no damage to his heart. He was back at work within several days, later resumed full exercise capacity and is again working with trying to take statins at the highest possible dose that doesn't cause side-effects. We are continuing with follow-up stress testing.

All this has occurred with an inflexible and difficult response by his insurance company. Yet his management, I believe, has been a model of what can be possible if we know what is going on in the arteries and can be ahead of the game. I would argue, given his risk is now actually reduced because he was identified and treated appropriately, that his premium should have been adjusted down, not up! Imagine receiving a letter from your insurance company thanking you for being proactive and reducing your own risk – and by the way we will reduce your premium in line with this.

I've not provided an example but the same holds for licensing bodies and health checks for remote work location, fire fighters, service personnel, truck drivers and, of course, private and commercial pilots.

Change is needed – across the spectrum of related interests.

This change and the other departures considered throughout this book will be brought about by conversation followed by action. Many conversations will be had by all manner of people – specialists, GPs, patients and interested onlookers – who will share ideas, explore further and learn from one another. We will listen as well as talk and we will appreciate the difference and the opportunities. To be transformative, our conversations need to be open-ended, collaborative and reflective, and it will take time. Firstly, though, it needs a catalyst. Hence, this book, your readership and my invitation to you to be part of the conversation.

IMPORTANT POINTS

- This book is the beginning of a conversation, in which you are invited to participate.

- My vision is that:

  » CT imaging will be incorporated into an holistic preventative approach to coronary artery disease;

  » imaging findings will modify government-supported statin prescriptions;

  » public screening will become widespread so that precise, individualised care will be commonplace;

  » greater understanding of the underlying process of coronary atheroma will develop leading to now-only-imagined treatment possibilities, and

  » insurance and other regulatory bodies will take a more proactive and less prescriptive view to people with plaque in their arteries.

[1]   Achenbach S, Ropers D, Pohle K, et al. Influence of Lipid-Lowering Therapy on the Progression of Coronary Artery Calcification: A Prospective Evaluation. Circulation 2002;106:1077-82.

[2]   Raggi P, Callister TQ, Shaw LJ. Progression of coronary artery calcium and risk of first myocardial infarction in patients receiving cholesterol-lowering therapy. Arterioscler Thromb Vasc Biol 2004;24:1272-7.

Epilogue

I have an enthusiasm about, and belief in, the technology of cardiac CT and what it can offer, tempered with an understanding of some of the hurdles preventing it from being more broadly used. From a practical as well as a logical perspective, cardiac CT imaging's contribution to improved patient care is markedly under-utilised.

The deficiency in supportive data from randomised controlled trials means that my colleagues, specifically cardiology specialists who could lead change in clinical management, are not comfortable in using the technology due to the lack of an appropriate evidence base. This scepticism can flow to general practitioners who are unlikely to unilaterally embrace a technology that does not appear to have the backing of the specialist group responsible for that area of medicine.

In focussing a spotlight on a technology that could be more widely used for the benefit of individuals and, subsequently, larger communities, I believe this book demonstrates that there is ample observational data available to support the uptake of the technology and provide guidance in the first instance. At no stage has it been my intention to diminish the importance of evidence-based medicine as the guide to how medicine decides on the direction of ongoing care. However, I believe that evidenced-based medicine should create the foundations of good medicine, not erect immoveable boundaries.

I am prepared to wear any criticism that will come my way from my evidence-based-only colleagues as, until our understanding of medicine is complete, evidence cannot provide all the answers. Nuances and variability within a circumstance, and clinical experience together with patient choice, need to be considered for good medicine to be practised.

What I also realised was that the person most interested in being aware of what is available is the patient: **YOU!** This book has been written specifically to provide information which will allow you, should you be a patient, to engage with your general practitioner and your specialist in a more detailed and robust exchange around what screening, treatment and/or management might be appropriate for you.

Criticism and controversy are healthy parts of vigorous conversation, as too, are vision, passion and an enthusiasm for possibility. If this book starts such conversation that opens doors to further evaluation, consideration and discussion – and along the way improves medicine and saves lives – then that is a good start.

Wishing you good health.

Dr Warrick Bishop

Hobart, Tasmania, Australia

August 2016

Dr Bishop is available for medical and business consultancy and for speaking engagements. **Enquiries:** *warrick@drwarrickbishop.com*

Further copies of this book:
www.haveyouplannedyourheartattack.com.au

Appendix 1

What comes before coronary artery disease?
Defining atheroma burden

WARRICK BISHOP MB BS, FRACP

Recent advances in several technologies, such as CT imaging and intravascular ultrasound, allow evaluation of atheroma build up in the coronary arteries. The ability to provide images showing the extent of plaque formation within the coronary arteries before disorder of function is new to the management of coronary artery disease and perhaps consideration of new terminology is now required.

Key points

- **New technologies allow visualisation of coronary atheroma.**
- **Not all coronary atheroma will necessarily be high risk or cause a problem.**
- **Describing atheroma burden as coronary disease before symptoms or loss of function may not always be most appropriate.**
- **Defining atheroma burden may allow intervention to prevent development of disease.**

CARDIOLOGY TODAY 2015; 5(2): 22-24

Dr Bishop is a Cardiologist at Calvary Lenah Valley Hospital, Hobart, Tas. He has a strong interest in cardiac CT imaging, lipids and prevention.

istorically, coronary artery disease has been defined by the presence of symptoms, including angina, shortness of breath and acute coronary syndromes. This is because previously there has not been a means to evaluate the presence of plaque within the arteries of a well person until it impairs normal functioning with signs and symptoms or it is a 'disease state'.

Recent years have seen the development in several technologies, such as cardiac CT imaging, intravascular ultrasound, intra-coronary optical coherence tomography and magnetic resonance imaging, that allow evaluation of atheroma build up in the coronary arteries. Cardiac CT technology has become the most widespread and accessible.

Cardiac CT imaging can be performed without contrast (coronary calcium scan [CCS]) or with contrast (computed coronary tomography angiography [CCTA]). A detailed description of CCS and CCTA is beyond the scope of this article (for further details see: 'Coronary calcium scan and CT angiography: chalk and cheese' published in the September 2011 issue of *Cardiology Today*).[1] The importance of CCS and CCTA lie in their ability to provide images that evaluate plaque within the coronary arteries before a disorder of function or symptom. This is a situation that is new to the management of coronary artery disease and one that perhaps requires consideration of new terminology.

© PHOTOTAKE/KEVIN A. SOMERVILLE/DIOMEDIA.COM

Permission granted by Cardiology Today/MedicineToday for use in 'Have You Planned Your Heart Attack', by W. Bishop; for educational purposes © Medicine Today 2015

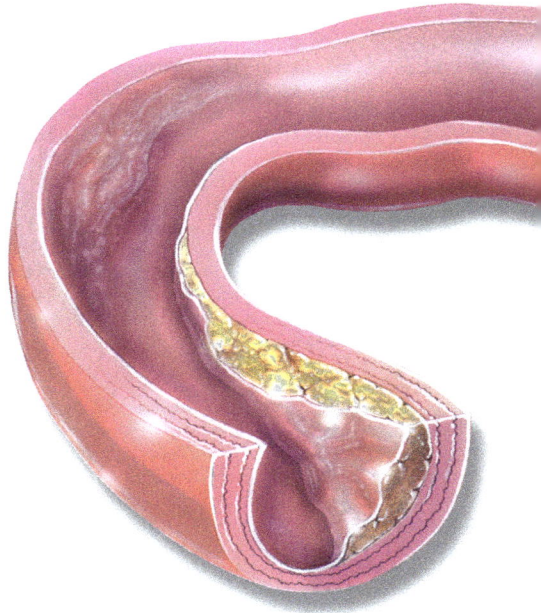

Why should we use the term atheroma burden?

In case 12 of the case study article in the September 2014 issue of *Cardiology Today*, the situation of finding plaque formation on cardiac CT imaging in a patient who presented in a primary prevention capacity (risk stratification) and had not had an event nor any symptom is presented.[2] This is someone who is otherwise healthy and was subsequently told he has coronary artery disease. In this situation, the term coronary artery disease may not be the most appropriate terminology to describe the situation. The patient felt and is well, and although he has plaque in his arteries, there is no disorder of function or symptom. A term that can be used for this situation is 'atheroma burden'. Reasons why we should use this term are discussed in more detail below.

There is not yet a disease

The patient described above has not yet had any event or symptom so the term 'disease' is not well received by the patient. It is much easier to have the conversation about 'a build up of cholesterol in the arteries that needs risk modification', rather than label the patient with a disease. There is a significant psychological cost in diagnosing a disease, particularly in a patient such as this who has presented in a primary prevention capacity feeling well. This type of patient is healthy and our objective is to keep them that way. This is the Holy Grail of preventive cardiology: to avoid the disease. Not using the term 'disease' requires the treating clinician to convey appropriately the risk of an event the patient may carry. There is no value in using more palatable terminology at the expense of complacency in management.

It can describe a spectrum

Atheroma burden is a term that allows interpretation along a spectrum of both the amount of atheroma and clinical setting. Compare two 60-year-old asymptomatic men, the first with a CCS score of 1 and the second with a CCS score of 1000. The first man has low-risk atheroma burden, whereas the second man has high-risk atheroma burden. They each require different management, so to label both men as having coronary disease fails to recognise the significant differences.

Compare an asymptomatic 70-year-old man with a CCS score of 50 and an asymptomatic 40-year-old woman with a CCS score of 50. They both have an equivalent amount of plaque burden based on the same score. In absolute terms the score is not particularly high and would likely carry a low risk of a cardiovascular event over the next 10 years.[3] For the 70-year-old man, this is a mild or low-risk atheroma burden for his age and sex[4,5] (below the 50th percentile) and unlikely to imply a significant change in the interpretation of risk from the CCS score alone. For the woman this is very high atheroma burden compared with an age- and sex-matched population[4,5] (greater than 90th percentile) and is likely to imply a significant change in the interpretation of the risk from the CCS score alone. It is a 'concerning atheroma burden' or 'potentially high-risk atheroma burden' and likely to represent a significant increase in lifetime risk of a cardiovascular event for this individual.[4,5]

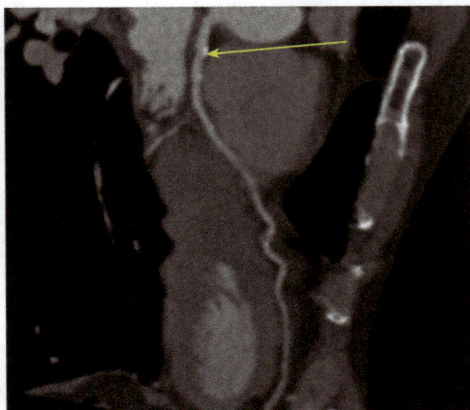

Figure. Computed coronary tomography angiography image of a coronary artery demonstrating proximal calcific plaque (arrow).

It is part of the ageing process

Lastly, development of atheroma in the coronary arteries appears part of the ageing process, such that if we were all to live long enough, we would all have evidence of wear and tear, or atheroma. The fact that this occurs more rapidly in some and more slowly in others simply reflects a different predisposition and not more or less aggressive disease, at least in the early stages, unless we wish to call the ageing process a disease. The term 'atheroma burden' allows description of a process that can progress at different rates in different individuals, as one might see in a patient with early joint degenerative change who does not yet have arthritic disease.

By recognising that the development of atheroma burden may be part of an ageing process, such that everyone will develop some, to some degree, with individual variation, creates the possibility that a change to terminology could improve the handling of patients such as the one described in case study 12.[2] This becomes important in the setting of life insurance or licensing as a pilot or commercial vehicle driver. High-risk atheroma burden or low-risk atheroma burden is a more valuable descriptor in this context compared with presence of plaque and therefore coronary artery disease.

Further discussion with case examples

A case example may help to illustrate the above. A 55-year-old man who is a commercial pilot presents with atypical chest pain and at low to intermediate risk of cardiovascular disease based on the results of a cardiovascular risk calculator. He undertakes cardiac CT imaging and his CCS score is 30 (see Figure). This shows low-risk atheroma burden for his age and sex (below the 50th percentile), without significant noncalcific plaque volume, remodelling or stenosis, features that have been observed to be linked to increasing risk. This is consistent with the predication from the cardiovascular risk

Permission granted by Cardiology Today/MedicineToday for use in 'Have You Planned Your Heart Attack', by W. Bishop; for educational purposes © Medicine Today 2015

calculator. If this patient were to have his pilot license threatened or have an increase in his health insurance premium because the presence of coronary calcium means he has been labelled as having coronary artery disease, then this misses the point because his cardiovascular disease risk is less than 5% over the next five years based just on the CCS score alone.[3] Of course other risk factors have to be considered to make a comprehensive clinical risk assessment. In this case, however, the features from imaging support the risk calculation from the cardiovascular risk calculator. Using the term 'coronary artery disease' seems not only inaccurate and clumsy but also detrimental to understanding the process.

Conversely, if we can take a healthy patient, who may have a high-risk atheroma burden, and reduce their risk of a cardiovascular event through appropriate intervention, then this would be good for everyone. In this setting, appropriate risk modification could avert an event or the disease. (Could it even justify reduced insurance premiums?)

Atheroma burden can allow a spectrum of significance and can be dealt with far more effectively than if we take a well patient and simply label them with a disease. A changing technology has changed the way we can evaluate the build up of cholesterol in the arteries. It would seem reasonable that we explore how terminology may need to move forward to fit with these changes.

A move towards using the term atheroma burden in clinical practice

Coronary atheroma burden may be defined as the extent of plaque formation in the coronary arteries as demonstrated on imaging before the development of disease. Coronary atheroma burden is not a new term, existing in the imaging lexicon, but it is perhaps time for it to become part of the clinical vernacular.

A move towards the use of the term 'coronary atheroma burden' in clinical practice requires description of potential risk-related features demonstrated on imaging. For cardiac CT imaging, this would include features such as the absolute CCS score, CCS percentile, plaque features including composition, remodelling, stenosis and location, described in a way to acknowledge the potential risk that the atheroma burden may represent.   CT

References
1. Hamilton-Craig, C, Hamilton-Craig I. Coronary calcium scan and CT angiography: chalk and cheese. Cardiology Today 2011; 1(3): 9-16.
2. Simons LA. Challenging cases in lipid management and CVD prevention. A retrospective and an update. Cardiology Today 2014; 4(3): 29-33.
3. Malik S, Budoff MJ, Katz R, et al. Impact of subclinical atherosclerosis on cardiovascular disease events in individuals with metabolic syndrome and diabetes: the multi-ethnic study of atherosclerosis. Diabetes Care 2011; 34: 2285-2290.
4. Wong ND, Budoff MJ, Pio J, Detrano RC. Coronary calcium and cardiovascular event risk: evaluation by age- and sex-specific quartiles. Am Heart J 2002; 143: 456-459.
5. Raggi P, Callister TQ, Cooil B, et al. Identification of patients at increased risk of first unheralded acute myocardial infarction by electron-beam computed tomography. Circulation 2000; 101: 850-855.

COMPETING INTERESTS: Dr Bishop has a financial and professional association with the iMed HeartView Cardiac CT service.

Permission granted by Cardiology Today/MedicineToday for use in 'Have You Planned Your Heart Attack', by W. Bishop; for educational purposes © Medicine Today 2015

Appendix 2

Describing the risk demonstrated on cardiac CT imaging
The C-PLUSS approach

WARRICK BISHOP MB BS, FRACP
MATTHEW BUDOFF MD

The C-PLUSS approach can be used to describe the risk-related features demonstrated on cardiac CT imaging. This approach incorporates features relating to coronary calcium together with plaque and vessel specific features, which have been shown to relate to cardiovascular risk. A descriptive risk comment, as part of the cardiac CT report, can then be generated, helping the referring clinician to understand their patient's potential future risks and so provide optimal care.

Key points

- Coronary calcium scoring is used predominately for risk assessment.
- Computed coronary tomography angiography is used predominately for the assessment of stenosis.
- Together, cardiac CT provides a snap shot of the health of the arteries.
- Different features seen within the arteries have been shown to be associated with future risk.
- Describing these features in combination may help future patient management.

CARDIOLOGY TODAY 2015; 5(3): 23-25

Dr Bishop is a Cardiologist at Calvary Lenah Valley Hospital, Hobart, Tas.
He has a strong interest in cardiac CT imaging, lipids and prevention.
Professor Budoff is a Professor of Medicine at Los Angeles Biomedical
Research Institute, California, USA.

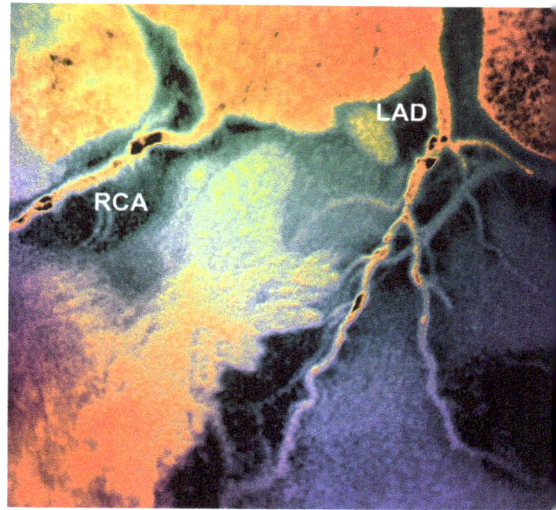

Risk-related features demonstrated on cardiac CT imaging are not reported in a structured way. In 1990 Agatston and colleagues developed the coronary calcium score (CCS),[1] and extensive work since has shown it to be a reproducible discriminator of cardiovascular risk that can be incorporated with standard Framingham-type risk calculation.[2,3] Findings on computed coronary tomography angiography (CCTA) that may impact risk, such as stenosis, noncalcific plaque and remodelling, have been linked with increased rates of a major adverse coronary event (MACE).[4-6] These observations open the possibility of incorporating these features into a risk comment, which combines both the CCS and CCTA findings, as part of the cardiac CT report. Factors that have a bearing on cardiovascular risk include:

- Calcium score
- calcium score Percentile
- Low attenuation plaque (LAP)
- Unfavourable remodelling
- Stenosis
- Site of plaque.

With observational risk data to support each of the above, these features can be incorporated and applied in the 'C-PLUSS' approach.

The C-PLUSS approach
Calcium scoring

A zero CCS in an asymptomatic individual is a powerful negative predictor of a MACE, and CCS alone has been shown reproducibly to be a discriminator of rates of a MACE in longitudinal studies.[1,2,7-10] CCS has also been shown to be the most reliable of the novel cardiovascular risk markers and, importantly, to improve risk stratification in the intermediate-risk patient group.[8,11] Increasing CCS is linked with increasing event rates and compared with standard Framingham-type risk models, CCS adds significant improvement and accuracy in risk assessment, even in people with prediabetes and diabetes.[3,8,9,11,12]

Percentile calcium score

For age and sex, the percentile calcium score has been documented to be linked to the likelihood of a MACE with the higher the percentile,

SEPTEMBER 2015, VOLUME 5, NUMBER 3   **CardiologyToday 23**

Permission granted by Cardiology Today/MedicineToday for use in 'Have You Planned Your Heart Attack', by W. Bishop; for educational purposes © Medicine Today 2015

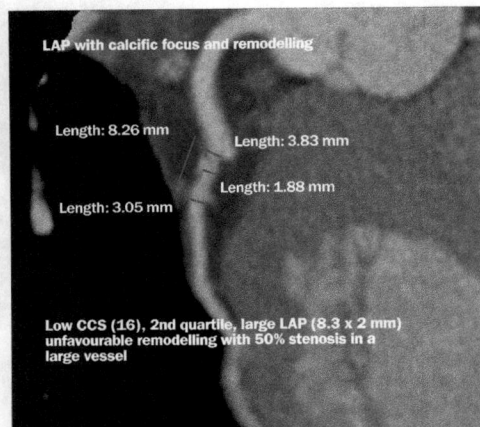

LAP with calcific focus and remodelling

Length: 8.26 mm

Length: 3.83 mm

Length: 3.05 mm

Length: 1.88 mm

Low CCS (16), 2nd quartile, large LAP (8.3 x 2 mm) unfavourable remodelling with 50% stenosis in a large vessel

Figure. Proximal left anterior descending (LAD) lesion with high-risk features greater than the coronary calcium score (CCS).
The following is an example of C-PLUSS risk comment of the lesion in the Figure above. LAD artery shows proximal calcific and noncalcific plaque, not flow limiting. The CCS of 16 and CCS percentile for age (2nd quartile) have been observed to be low-risk features, the presence of significant low attenuation plaque (LAP) burden with unfavourable remodelling has been observed to be associated with event rates of up to 20% in two   years. T hese are very high-risk features. The presence of a luminal narrowing of 50% or greater has been observed to be associated with event rates of up to 5% per annum. This is a very high-risk feature. The location of proximal LAD plaque defines a large territory potentially affected by an event. The features of this cardiac CT study have been observed to be a high to very high cardiovascular risk (>>20% risk in 10   years), with a large territory potentially affected. This information should be combined with an evaluation of the patient's other cardiovascular risks for a comprehensive risk profile to help in guiding further management.

the higher the risk.[13] The percentile calcium score is representative of a propensity for atheroma accumulation in an individual compared with an age- and sex-matched distribution, perhaps pointing to an increased lifetime risk. Wong and colleagues demonstrated an increased relative risk of approximately 3.5 for patients in the 3rd quartile and approximately 5.5 for patients in the 4th quartile compared with those in the first quartile of calcium scores.[10]

Low attenuation plaque and noncalcific plaque
LAP with a greater lipid core carries a higher risk of a coronary event than plaque that does not.[14-16] LAP assessment by CCTA has been validated by intravascular ultrasound.[17] Hoffman and colleagues documented that features of increasing LAP volume are linked to an increased rate of coronary events.[4-6,18] It has been observed that the presence of atherosclerotic lesions with a LAP volume of 20 mm³ or more (approximating LAP >8 mm x 2 mm) together with positive remodelling is a very high-risk feature.[5] Conversely, the relative

stability of calcific plaque without noncalcific plaque has also been suggested as a low-risk feature.[5] This suggests a spectrum of increasing risk as LAP volume and proportion within a particular plaque increases.[19] Furthermore, the presence of spotty calcification in LAP is linked to increased risk of a MACE and should be reported.[20,21] In the same way, reporting of the 'napkin-ring' sign, representing thin-cap fibroatheroma associated with a LAP burden, warrants description as a high-risk feature.[22,23]

Unfavourable remodelling
Positive, expansive or glagovian remodelling is the process in which the vessel changes shape (enlarges) to accommodate build up of atheroma within the wall, initially without encroachment on the lumen. This was first described by Glagov who suspected its unfavourable significance from autopsy, and subsequently this has been confirmed to be linked to an increased risk of a MACE.[24,25] Work carried out by Hoffman and colleagues showed the development of positive remodelling being linked to an increased rate of coronary events.[4-6] This has been quantified such that the presence of atherosclerotic lesions with remodelling of greater than 10% (remodelled artery diameter 10% increased) can be associated with a 3.5% event rate in two years.[5]

Although the accepted term is 'positive remodelling', 'unfavourable remodelling' is a deliberate and practical nomenclature to avoid possible ambiguity that could arise with the term 'positive'. 'Unfavourable' is a descriptor to assist the clinician who may not be familiar with cardiac CT terminology and the increased risk 'positive remodelling' can carry (see Figure).

Stenosis
In the coronary arteries, the degree of stenosis has been linked to rates of a coronary event, the more severe the stenosis, the higher the event rate.[26] CCTA has supported this finding in the Coronary CT Angiography Evaluation For Clinical Outcomes: an International Multicenter (CONFIRM) registry and recent data have suggested luminal narrowing of 50% or more is linked to event rates of over 5% per annum.[6,27,28]

Site of plaque (location)
The site of plaque is described as part of the anatomical assessment of a CCTA; however, it also has significance in regard to prognostication. An event related to plaque rupture in a proximal large vessel supplying a significant territory of myocardium is an important distinction from a similar quality plaque in a distal location supplying a small territory because infarct size and postinfarction left ventricular volume are linked to outcome.[29-31] There is prognostic significance in recognising potential myocardial territory at risk from a specific plaque. Knowing proximal large vessel plaque compared with distally located plaque in a small vessel may give the treating physician more information in choosing the most appropriate therapy for example in a patient having difficulty achieving lipid targets.

Permission granted by Cardiology Today/MedicineToday for use in 'Have You Planned Your Heart Attack', by W. Bishop; for educational purposes © Medicine Today 2015

What do the results of the C-PLUSS model tell you?

In the C-PLUSS approach, the calcium score is used as the basis of risk assessment. Each subsequent factor is then assessed as either having no significant effect on the CCS risk assessment or having an upregulating effect on the CCS risk assessment. A descriptive risk comment can be generated (see Table), thus providing a structure to interpreting the risk-related features. The reader or reporter of the scan can then incorporate the available data to best fit the findings, therefore providing a conclusion that is complimentary to standard risk calculation with low, intermediate, high and very high risk features (representing <10%, 10–20%, >20% and >>20% 10-year risk of a MACE, respectively). This information can then be used as an adjunct to standard risk assessment. It should not be considered as a replacement for existing risk modelling based on Framingham-type calculators.

An example of how the C-PLUSS model aids in dealing with patient risk based on the CCS and how this may require adjustment based on lesion-specific findings is shown in the Figure. Combining the C-PLUSS conclusion with an evaluation of standard risk factors for the patient is mandatory because the cardiac CT represents one moment in time and other risk factors the future. The clinician therefore needs to comprehensively bring all this information together to achieve optimal patient care.

Objective of the C-PLUSS approach

The objective of the C-PLUSS approach is to provide a structure for describing cardiac CT features that have been shown to relate to risk. It is intended to use the CCS as a basis for risk assessment then allow description of the 'PLUSS' findings by the reader or reporter of the study who can then provide an experienced, educated and informed comment on the risk features demonstrated by the cardiac CT. There will always be a spectrum of risk findings that will need interpretation because exact details will not exist. It is then the role of the treating physician to assess all risk factors of the patient to best plan management. Some patients may undergo CCS scoring without CCTA, and some may undergo CCTA without CCS. This is a decision of the local service or referrer. Using both however will provide the most information to aid in risk evaluation.

Table. Summary of C-PLUSS features and associated risk of a major adverse coronary event

C-PLUSS feature	Magnitude	Risk level
CCS	<50	Low
	50 to 400	Intermediate
	>400	High
CCS percentile	>3rd quartile	Upregulates CCS risk by up to threefold, and increases lifetime risk
	>4th quartile	Upregulates CCS risk by up to fourfold, and increases lifetime risk
LAP volume (<30 Hounsfield units) spectrum	Calcium >> LAP (ratio)	May not further increase risk significantly
	Calcium = LAP (ratio)	May further increase risk
	LAP >> calcium (ratio)	Likely to further increase risk
Significant LAP with or without napkin-ring sign	>2 x 8 mm lesion Volume approx >20 mm³	High risk (up to 5% event rate in two years or > 25% in 10 years)
Unfavourable remodelling	>10% increase in diameter	High risk (up to 5% event rate in two years or > 25% in 10 years)
Significant LAP with or without napkin-ring sign and unfavourable remodelling	Soft plaque >2 x 8 mm lesion Plus >10% increase in diameter	Very high risk (up to 20% event rate in two years or approaching 100% in 10 years)
Stenosis	>50%	Very high risk (event rates of 5% or more per annum or >50% in 10 years)
Site	Major/minor artery, proximal or distal plaque	Comment on amount of territory at risk

Abbreviations: CCS = coronary calcium score; LAP = low attenuation plaque.

Using the C-PLUSS approach in clinical practice

Despite the absence of outcome data, the C-PLUSS approach will be driven by clinicians wanting to incorporate as much information as possible to achieve the best assessment and care for their patients. A risk comment would help the General Practitioner who refers patients for nonrebatable risk assessment, and who receives reports from patients who have had a rebatable scan. Clinicians could ask their local cardiac CT service to provide a C-PLUSS comment. Using CCS as the first step of risk assessment, the C-PLUSS approach aims to facilitate a reproducible way to describe the risk-related features demonstrated on cardiac CT imaging. **CT**

References

A list of references is included in the website version (www.medicinetoday.com.au) of this article.

COMPETING INTERESTS: Dr Bishop has a financial and professional association with the iMed HeartView Cardiac CT service. Professor Budoff is a Research Consultant for General Electric Company.

Permission granted by Cardiology Today/MedicineToday for use in 'Have You Planned Your Heart Attack', by W. Bishop; for educational purposes © Medicine Today 2015

Describing the risk demonstrated on cardiac CT imaging
The C-PLUSS approach

WARRICK BISHOP MB BS, FRACP; **MATTHEW BUDOFF** MD

References

1. Agatston AS, Janowitz WR, Hildner FJ, Zusmer NR, Viamonte M, Jr, Detrano R. Quantification of coronary artery calcium using ultrafast computed tomography. J Am Coll Cardiol 1990; 15: 827-832.

2. Greenland P, Bonow RO, Brundage BH, et al. ACCF/AHA 2007 clinical expert consensus document on coronary artery calcium scoring by computed tomography in global cardiovascular risk assessment and in evaluation of patients with chest pain: a report of the American College of Cardiology Foundation Clinical Expert Consensus Task Force (ACCF/AHA Writing Committee to Update the 2000 Expert Consensus Document on Electron Beam Computed Tomography). Circulation 2007; 115: 402-426.

3. Malik S, Budoff MJ, Katz R, et al. Impact of subclinical atherosclerosis on cardiovascular disease events in individuals with metabolic syndrome and diabetes: the multi-ethnic study of atherosclerosis. Diabetes Care 2011; 34: 2285-2290.

4. Hoffmann U, Moselewski F, Nieman K, et al. Noninvasive assessment of plaque morphology and composition in culprit and stable lesions in acute coronary syndrome and stable lesions in stable angina by multidetector computed tomography. J Am Coll Cardiol 2006; 47: 1655-1662.

5. Motoyama S, Sarai M, Harigaya H, et al. Computed tomographic angiography characteristics of atherosclerotic plaques subsequently resulting in acute coronary syndrome. J Am Coll Cardiol 2009; 54: 49-57.

6. Yamamoto H, Kitagawa T, Ohashi N, et al. Noncalcified atherosclerotic lesions with vulnerable characteristics detected by coronary CT angiography and future coronary events. J Cardiovasc Comput Tomogr 2013; 7: 192-199.

7. Sarwar A, Shaw LJ, Shapiro MD, et al. Diagnostic and prognostic value of absence of coronary artery calcification. JACC Cardiovasc Imaging 2009; 2: 675-688.

8. Yeboah J, McClelland RL, Polonsky TS, et al. Comparison of novel risk markers for improvement in cardiovascular risk assessment in intermediate-risk individuals. JAMA 2012; 308: 788-795.

9. Budoff MJ, Shaw LJ, Liu ST, et al. Long-term prognosis associated with coronary calcification: observations from a registry of 25,253 patients. J Am Coll Cardiol 2007; 49: 1860-1870.

10. Wong ND, Budoff MJ, Pio J, Detrano RC. Coronary calcium and cardiovascular event risk: evaluation by age- and sex-specific quartiles. Am Heart J 2002; 143: 456-459.

11. Elias-Smale SE, Proenca RV, Koller MT, et al. Coronary calcium score improves classification of coronary heart disease risk in the elderly: the Rotterdam study. J Am Coll Cardiol 2010; 56: 1407-1414.

12. LaMonte MJ, FitzGerald SJ, Church TS, et al. Coronary artery calcium score and coronary heart disease events in a large cohort of asymptomatic men and women. Am J Epidemiol 2005; 162: 421-429.

13. Raggi P, Callister TQ, Cooil B, et al. Identification of patients at increased risk of first unheralded acute myocardial infarction by electron-beam computed tomography. Circulation 2000; 101: 850-855.

14. Falk E, Shah PK, Fuster V. Coronary plaque disruption. Circulation 1995; 92: 657-671.

15. Matsumoto N, Sato Y, Yoda S, et al. Prognostic value of non-obstructive CT low-dense coronary artery plaques detected by multislice computed tomography. Circ J 2007; 71: 1898-1903.

16. Komatsu S, Imai A, Kodama K. Multidetector row computed tomography may accurately estimate plaque vulnerability: does MDCT accurately estimate plaque vulnerability? (Pro). Circ J 2011; 75: 1515-1521.

17. Motoyama S, Kondo T, Anno H, et al. Atherosclerotic plaque characterization by 0.5-mm-slice multislice computed tomographic imaging. Circ J 2007; 71: 363-366.

18. Versteylen MO, Kietselaer BL, Dagnelie PC, et al. Additive value of semiautomated quantification of coronary artery disease using cardiac computed tomographic angiography to predict future acute coronary syndrome. J Am Coll Cardiol 2013; 61: 2296-2305.

19. Kristensen TS, Kofoed KF, Kuhl JT, Nielsen WB, Nielsen MB, Kelbaek H. Prognostic implications of nonobstructive coronary plaques in patients with non-ST-segment elevation myocardial infarction: a multidetector computed tomography study. J Am Coll Cardiol 2011; 58: 502-509.

20. Ehara S, Kobayashi Y, Yoshiyama M, et al. Spotty calcification typifies the culprit plaque in patients with acute myocardial infarction: an intravascular ultrasound study. Circulation 2004; 110: 3424-3429.

21. van Velzen JE, de Graaf FR, de Graaf MA, et al. Comprehensive assessment of spotty calcifications on computed tomography angiography: comparison to plaque characteristics on intravascular ultrasound with radiofrequency backscatter analysis. J Nucl Cardiol 2011; 18: 893-903.

22. Kashiwagi M, Tanaka A, Kitabata H, et al. Feasibility of noninvasive assessment of thin-cap fibroatheroma by multidetector computed tomography. JACC Cardiovasc Imaging 2009; 2: 1412-1419.

23. Narula J, Achenbach S. Napkin-ring necrotic cores: defining circumferential extent of necrotic cores in unstable plaques: JACC Cardiovasc Imaging 2009; 2: 1436-1438.

24. Glagov S, Weisenberg E, Zarins CK, Stankunavicius R, Kolettis GJ. Compensatory enlargement of human atherosclerotic coronary arteries. N Engl J Med 1987; 316: 1371-1375.

25. Varnava AM, Mills PG, Davies MJ. Relationship between coronary artery remodeling and plaque vulnerability. Circulation 2002; 105: 939-943.

26. Harris PJ, Behar VS, Conley MJ, et al. The prognostic significance of 50% coronary stenosis in medically treated patients with coronary artery disease. Circulation 1980; 62: 240-248.

27. Min JK, Dunning A, Lin FY, et al. Age- and sex-related differences in all-cause mortality risk based on coronary computed tomography angiography findings results from the International Multicenter CONFIRM (Coronary CT Angiography evaluation for clinical outcomes: an international Multicenter Registry) of 23,854 patients without known coronary artery disease. J Am Coll Cardiol 2011; 58: 849-860.

28. Hulten EA, Carbonaro S, Petrillo SP, Mitchell JD, Villines TC. Prognostic value of cardiac computed tomography angiography: a systematic review and meta-analysis. J Am Coll Cardiol 2011; 57: 1237-1247.

29. Watts GF, Sullivan DR, Poplawski N, et al. Familial hypercholesterolaemia: a model of care for Australasia. Atheroscler Suppl 2011; 12: 221-263.

30. Arno PS, Viola D. Hypertension treatment at the crossroads: a role for economics? Am J Hypertens 2013; 26: 1257-1259.

31. Wang G, Yan L, Ayala C, George MG, Fang J. Hypertension-associated expenditures for medication among US adults. Am J Hypertens 2013; 26: 1295-1302.

Permission granted by Cardiology Today/MedicineToday for use in 'Have You Planned Your Heart Attack', by W. Bishop; for educational purposes © Medicine Today 2015

Appendix 3

My suggested cardiac CT user guide for Australian General Practitioners

Following rapid development in recent years, cardiac CT imaging is now widely available. There are two components to cardiac CT imaging: firstly, coronary artery calcium (CAC), a non-contrast set of images, and secondly, there is coronary computed tomography angiography (CCTA) which requires injection of contrast to detail the arteries. CAC is the descriptor for the presence of calcium in the arteries; coronary calcium score (CCS) quantifies the calcium. Calcium as a marker of atherosclerotic plaque within the arteries has been well established as correlating to cardiovascular (CV) risk of events[1-5]. The term, CAC, is often used interchangeably with CCS. CCTA is a contrast acquisition study and demonstrates anatomical detail of the coronary arteries for assessment of potential stenosis but also demonstrates features of plaque morphology[6-8].

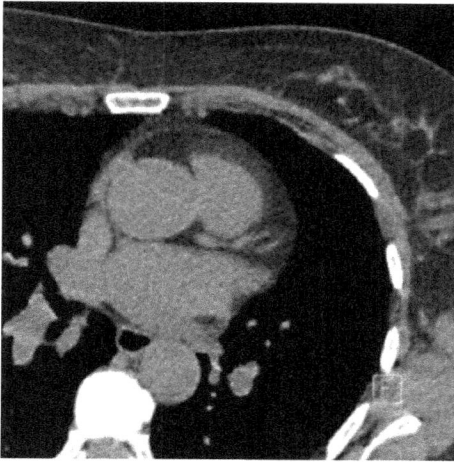

Non-contrast CAC.

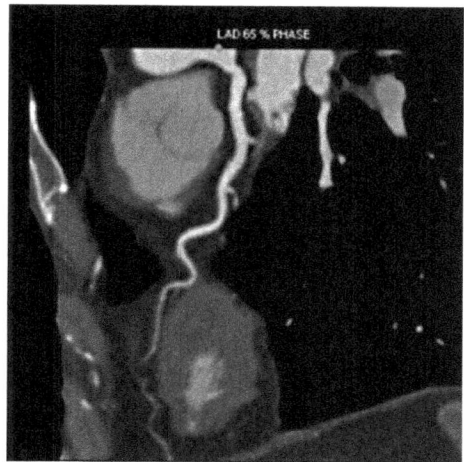

Contrast used for CCTA.

There are two groups of patients who may be considered for CT imaging of the heart. The first group is symptomatic patients for whom imaging would be used for evaluation of possible coronary stenosis. The second group consists of asymptomatic patients and CT imaging would be used for risk evaluation.

Currently in Australia a rebate exists for CCTA, requested by a specialist as per item 57360:

Computed Tomography of the Coronary Arteries performed on a minimum of a 64 slice (or equivalent) scanner, when the request is made by a specialist or consultant physician, and:

a) the patient has stable symptoms consistent with coronary ischaemia, is at low to intermediate risk of coronary artery disease and would have been considered for coronary angiography, or

b) the patient requires exclusion of coronary artery anomaly or fistula, or

c) the patient will be undergoing non-coronary cardiac surgery.

Fee: $700.00 Benefit: 75% = $525.00, 85% = $623.80

Currently in Australia there is no rebate for CAC (nor CCTA) for risk stratification, regardless of the referring doctor.

Assessment of symptoms

Rebatable

Depending on the clinical assessment of the reviewing specialist, below are a number situations in which CCTA may be utilised to evaluate the coronary arteries. Importantly, the requesting specialist will have to satisfy the questions "Is this patient low to intermediate risk of obstructive coronary disease?" **and** "Would this patient otherwise be a candidate for angiography?"

- Evaluation of possible cardiac symptoms with no previous known disease (clinic patient):
  » unable to exercise or ECG uninterpretable;
  » equivocal stress test results, or
  » normal stress test but recurrent or ongoing symptoms.

- Evaluation of possible acute coronary syndrome (emergency department patient):
  » normal ECG and cardiac enzymes, suggestive history, or
  » low-to-intermediate pre-test probability of CAD, suggestive history.
- Exclusion of CAD in new-onset heart failure/cardiomyopathy.
- Assessment of CABG patency.

A growing body of evidence supporting the use of CCTA for evaluation of stenosis[9] and for its utility in the accident and emergency setting[10,11] would suggest this technology will continue to see increased uptake.

Dealing with the results for the primary care physician

For the primary care physician there are a number of important points of understanding in dealing with the ongoing care of a patient who has had a CCTA. If there is a suspected stenosis, this will have been dealt with by the specialist who ordered the test. If, however, there is plaque demonstrated but no suggestion of stenosis, then the extent of the atheroma burden and the risk it may portend will be reflected in correspondence from the specialist who ordered the test, to help guide future risk management[12]. *(See Appendix 1 on atheroma burden and Appendix 2, C-PLUSS.)* The other important issue is to follow up on incidental findings, for example, lung nodules that may warrant follow-up surveillance scanning. Cardiopulmonary incidental findings (such as PE, PFO, ASD, VSD, anomalous pulmonary venous drainage, anomalous SVC, hypertrophic cardiomyopathy, LV thinning/previous infarction and possible cardiac tumours) will generally only be seen with CCTA and not CAC alone. The requesting specialist will deal with these findings as appropriate to the patient.

Assessment of cardiovascular risk in asymptomatic patients

Not rebatable

Both the European Society of Cardiology and the American College of Cardiology Foundation/American Heart Association have produced guidelines supporting the use of CAC for improving risk stratification in the intermediate-risk patient. The Cardiac Society of Australia and New Zealand has recently ratified a position statement.

The following situations may be circumstances when an improved understanding of a patient's coronary atheroma burden to refine risk assessment may help to achieve the best possible care for the patient.

1) *A patient with a high cholesterol, otherwise at intermediate risk, who does not want to take statin therapy.* "Do I really need to take a statin?"

2) *A patient with an unremarkable cholesterol profile but a strong positive family history of premature coronary disease.*
"All the men in my family died before they were 55 years old and I'm 54. Should I be worried?"

3) *A patient with intermediate risk but who has some risk factors, i.e. may be sedentary, recently gained weight, wants to be proactive, had a close friend recently die, and wishes to be evaluated.*
"A mate of mine dropped dead a month ago walking out of the gym. Could it happen to me?"

4) *A patient with high cholesterol and high cardiovascular risk features who may have mild intolerance of statins.* "I can take a bit but at higher doses I get aches and pains. Do I really need the higher dose or is there some other therapy?"

In these situations, a GP may find imaging a valuable aid to help in providing more information to guide discussion and decisions for management of the individual. With explanation and education, many patients are comfortable to pay for the testing ($300 or less in most centres for CAC) to be clear about the status of their own arteries to guide individualised management.

Understanding cardiac CT in risk evaluation

Cardiac CT allows precision around the actual health of the arteries of an individual compared with risk calculators, which provide an estimate of the likelihood of an event within a population which shares the same characteristics. For example, let's consider an individual patient who is male, 50 years old, with borderline blood pressure 135mmHg, mild cholesterol elevation 5.8mmol/l, HDL of 1.1 mmol/l, non-smoker, non-diabetic and no LVH on ECG; the rate of event (AUST RISK CALC) is 5% in 5 years. This is a rate that is not particularly high but if we were then to consider 100 men with the same calculated risk, five would have a major coronary event (MACE) in the next five years. If we scan the population, we will find there is a bell distribution curve of results, with some individuals in the group having high-to very high-risk features (those likely to have events in the next five years) and conversely, some demonstrating very low-risk features. CT imaging allows a **tailored approach** for the individual based on the **actual health** of that person's arteries compared with the **possible risk** as determined by a population. This becomes important as most risk calculators are heavily weighted for age and do not include factors such as family history, exercise, waist-to-hip ratio and pre-diabetic status, factors which may be of significance in the individual.

So, imaging offers information about the health of that person's arteries rather than the population in which that person finds him or herself. This aids in decision-making.

When and what to request

For male patients over 50 and female patients over 60, without symptoms and at calculated intermediate CV risk, request "coronary artery calcium score".

In my practice, I request CAC to progress to CCTA if the score is > zero. Although this is not a current guideline, I discuss my rationale earlier in the book.

For patients with significant lipid abnormality, family history of premature coronary artery disease, younger than 55 for a male or 60 for a female, consider referral to a cardiologist with an interest in imaging and prevention.

Before requesting testing, it is important to raise two issues with the patient. **Firstly,** that a patient at low to intermediate risk based on risk calculation may not fulfil the pharmaceutical benefits scheme criteria for prescription of statin therapy, even if the CAC demonstrates high-risk features. In this situation, the patient may be obliged to cover the full cost of the medication. **Secondly,** whatever the findings of the test, the results will need to be disclosed – to an insurance company, a regulatory authority or similar organisation. Here, I suggest patients seek professional advice in relation to what impact the result will have on policies or occupation.

Dealing with the results

In dealing with results:

- A zero **coronary calcium score** in an asymptomatic patient carries with it a very low risk (<1%) of event over the subsequent 10 years[13]. If calcium is present, then in absolute terms, the higher the score the greater the risk. An absolute score over 400 is considered a high-risk finding and over 1000, a very high-risk finding[2].

- The higher the **percentile** (how the score compares within 100 age and sex matched equivalents) the greater the lifetime risk that individual will carry. To understand the percentile, compare an asymptomatic 68-year-old male with a calcium score of 25 and an asymptomatic 38-year-old male with a calcium score of 25. They have an equivalent amount of plaque burden based on the same score. In absolute terms the score is not particularly high and would likely carry a low risk of event over the next 10 years[14]. For the 68-year-old, this is a 'mild or low atheroma burden' for age and sex[4,15] (less than 25th percentile, see nomogram red circle) and unlikely to imply a significant change in the interpretation of risk from the absolute CCS alone. For the younger man, this is 'very high atheroma burden' compared with an age and sex matched population[4,15] (greater than 90th percentile, see nomogram green circle) and is likely to imply a significant change in the interpretation of the risk from the CAC alone. It is a 'concerning atheroma burden' or 'potentially high-risk atheroma burden', and likely to represent a significant increase in CV events for this individual in the future[4,15].

So a zero CAC becomes more reliable the older the patient is. This is best understood by considering CAC nomograms. Looking at the table, the red rectangle shows how a zero calcium score may still be found in a 35-39-year-old male patient up to the 75th percentile, while the green rectangle shows how in a 50-54-year-old male patient, zero CAC falls within the 25th percentile.

Calcium score nomogram for 9728 consecutive subjects

AGE (Years)

	35–39	40–44	45–49	50–54	55–59	60–64	65–70
Men	(479)	(859)	(1066)	(1085)	(853)	(613)	(478)
25th percentile	0	0	0	0	3	14	28
50th percentile	0	0	3	16	41	118	151
75th percentile	2	11	44	101	187	434	569
90th percentile	21	64	176	320	502	804	1178
Women	(288)	(589)	(822)	(903)	(693)	(515)	(485)
25th percentile	0	0	0	0	0	0	0
50th percentile	0	0	0	0	0	4	24
75th percentile	0	0	0	10	33	87	123
90th percentile	4	9	23	66	140	310	362

A zero calcium score that also clearly puts the asymptomatic patient in the first quartile for age and sex (men 50 and older, and women 60 and older) is a very robust negative predictor of an event.

The Agatston Score evaluates the heart in 3mm slices (the slice thickness of the EBT scanner first used and on which the original work was done). Current generation multi-slice CT scanners can obtain 0.6mm slices, which increases the sensitivity of calcium detection such that a "zero" on 3mm slices may demonstrate "flecks" of calcification on 0.6mm slices[16].

For risk stratifying asymptomatic younger patients, a zero score may fall anywhere between the first and fourth quartiles. In this situation, fine cut 0.6mm slices/reconstructions may be utilised. This is a specialist area but nonetheless interesting in facilitating understanding of the technology.

Matching the results with the patient

The results of the CAC will generally be reported as a risk based on an absolute score plus or minus comment on percentile. This will provide CAC features that are low, intermediate or high risk. The referring physician will then need to decide on patient care based on a comprehensive clinical assessment. However, the following may guide a potential approach.

CAC "low-risk features"

In the setting of a low-risk factor profile, **nothing further to do.**

In the setting of an intermediate-risk factor profile, **lifestyle modification.**

Cardiac CT "intermediate-risk features"

In the setting of a low-risk factor profile, work on **lifestyle modification.**

In the setting of an intermediate-risk factor profile, manage as per **NDVPA guidelines**[17].

Cardiac CT "high-risk features"

In the setting of a low- to intermediate-risk factor profile, consider treating as **high risk.**

Cardiac CT "very high-risk features"

Consider **cardiologist review.**
In certain situations, **family screening** may be appropriate.

What if there is a very high calcium score (>90th percentile) or very high-risk features?

I would suggest referral to a cardiologist with an interest in preventative cardiology. High CCS can be associated with coronary artery stenosis and may warrant functional testing to be evaluated further[18]. Further testing may include insulin sensitivity, homocysteine levels, apo lipoprotein B, lipoprotein a and, in appropriate cases, family screening and screening for familial hypercholesterolemia.

What if there is a zero calcium score in a patient who seems to otherwise be at increased risk?

This patient should be treated as per the NVDPA guidelines as the possibility of CCS not representing possible non-calcified plaque burden needs to be considered *(see images below)*. This is why I use CCTA as part of a thorough risk assessment. Standard risk reduction/modification, such as weight loss and exercise, should still be undertaken[17]. This may be a situation to discuss with your local preventative cardiologist.

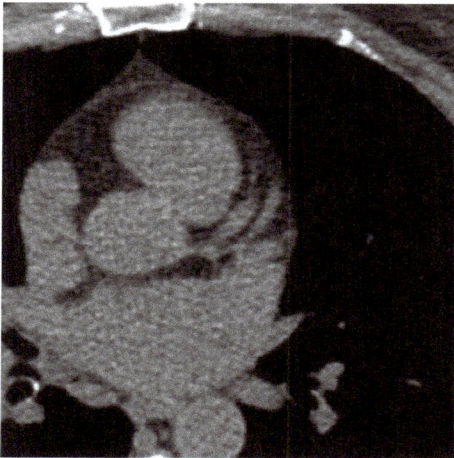

Occasional finding of low CCS.

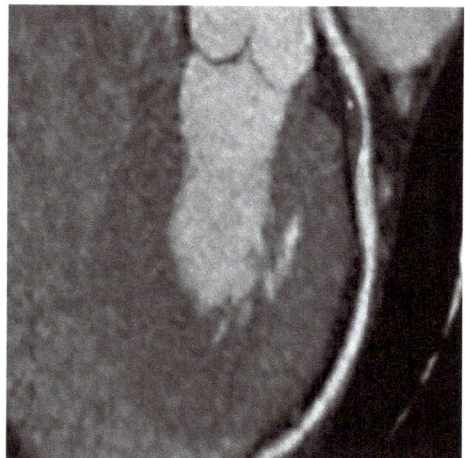

With high-risk non-calcific plaque.

Is there a role for repeat scanning?

Although some patients may ask, current literature **does not** support routine use of repeat scanning. However, there has been research into the rate of change of CCS per annum[19]. It suggests that a rate of change of CCS of >10-15% p.a. or an increase of an absolute score of more than 100 p.a. carries a significantly higher rate of event compared with a rate of change of <10-15% per annum. In selected patients, who perhaps have difficulty with compliance or in achieving targets, with specialist involvement, repeat CCS may be considered appropriate.

Preparation for cardiac CT: heart rate

Ideally, for cardiac CT, the heart rate should be less than 55 beats per minute.

If the heart rate control is inadequate, the pictures will be inadequate.

In most cases, beta-blockers are given to reduce the heart rate. I use a formatted preparation envelope[20]. The medication can be prescribed by script. However, I have a box of metoprolol with a pair of scissors in my drawer and cut a few off for the patient.

I suggest an ECG on all patients.

If on ECG the patient has normal sinus rhythm and no evidence of heart block, then I use the following as a guide, although different units may have their own protocol.

If the patient is already on a beta-blocker, an additional dose of the regular medication at 1.5 hours prior to the study is suggested, adjusted to the resting heart rate.

For a patient not currently on any cardiac medication and with a blood pressure greater than 110mmHg, having fully evaluated the patient, I use the following drug protocols. These protocols use relatively high doses. However, in my experience, these provide the best chance for optimal heart rate control.

Resting heart rate between 55 and 65,

> » metoprolol 50mg orally – **two** doses: 50mg the night before and 50mg 1.5 hours before the scan time.

Resting heart rate between 65 and 75,

> » metoprolol 50mg orally – **two** doses: 100mg the night before, and 100mg 1.5 hours before the scan time.

Resting heart rate between 75 and 85,

> » metoprolol 50mg orally – **three** doses: 100mg the night before, 100mg first thing the morning of the scan (0600) and 100mg 1.5 hours before the scan time.

Resting heart rate greater than 85,

> » consider specialist input.

For patients with **asthma** or on **calcium channel blockers,** diltiazem and verapamil, **beta-blockers should be avoided** to prevent drug interaction. For these patients and patients with complex medical histories, drug regimens or with rhythm disturbance AF, VEs, first or second degree heart block, consider referral to a cardiologist for assessment and safe, effective heart rate management.

Situations that warrant specialist review

RHYTHM DISTURBANCE, AF or MULTIPLE VEs: Irregular heartbeats will make image acquisition challenging for cardiac CT, leading to image degradation. Alternate evaluation may be indicated.

SYMPTOMS/PREVIOUS CAD: Specialist referral may lead to a rebatable scan or an alternate clinically appropriate evaluation.

Summary

Cardiac CT imaging is currently accessible with government rebate in Australia as an alternate to invasive coronary angiography, mainly for evaluation of symptoms for intermediate-risk patients. Although not rebatable for risk stratification, the test offers precision around the health of an individual's arteries and so potentially better defines that patient's risk. Many patients may wish to explore the improved risk stratification imaging can offer. It is important for general practitioners to be aware of the technology, the results it may provide and how it may aid in the care of their patients.

[1] Agatston AS, Janowitz WR, Hildner FJ, Zusmer NR, Viamonte JM, Detrano R. Quantification of coronary artery calcium using ultrafast computed tomography. J Am Coll Cardiol 1990;15:827-32.

[2] Greenland P, Bonow RO, Brundage BH, et al. ACCF/AHA 2007 clinical expert consensus document on coronary artery calcium scoring by computed tomography in global cardiovascular risk assessment and in evaluation of patients with chest pain: a report of the American College of Cardiology Foundation Clinical Expert Consensus Task Force (ACCF/AHA Writing Committee to Update the 2000 Expert Consensus Document on Electron Beam Computed Tomography) developed in collaboration with the Society of Atherosclerosis Imaging and Prevention and the Society of Cardiovascular Computed Tomography. J Am Coll Cardiol 2007;49: 378-402.

[3] Yeboah J, McClelland RL, Polonsky TS, et al. Comparison of novel risk markers for improvement in cardiovascular risk assessment in intermediate-risk individuals. Jama 2012;308:788-95.

[4] Wong ND, Budoff MJ, Pio J, Detrano RC. Coronary calcium and cardiovascular event risk: evaluation by age- and sex-specific quartiles. Am Heart J 2002;143:456-9.

[5] Budoff MJ, Shaw LJ, Liu ST, et al. Long-term prognosis associated with coronary calcification: observations from a registry of 25,253 patients. J Am Coll Cardiol 2007;49:1860-70.

[6] Hoffmann U, Moselewski F, Nieman K, et al. Noninvasive assessment of plaque morphology and composition in culprit and stable lesions in acute coronary syndrome and stable lesions in stable angina by multidetector computed tomography. J Am Coll Cardiol 2006;47:1655-62.

[7] Motoyama S, Sarai M, Harigaya H, et al. Computed tomographic angiography characteristics of atherosclerotic plaques subsequently resulting in acute coronary syndrome. J Am Coll Cardiol 2009;54:49-57.

[8]   Yamamoto H, Kitagawa T, Ohashi N, et al. Noncalcified atherosclerotic lesions with vulnerable characteristics detected by coronary CT angiography and future coronary events. Journal of cardiovascular computed tomography 2013;7:192-99.

[9]   Arbab-Zadeh A, Miller JM, Rochitte CE, et al. Diagnostic Accuracy of Computed Tomography Coronary Angiography According to Pre-Test Probability of Coronary Artery Disease and Severity of Coronary Arterial Calcification The CORE 64 (Coronary Artery Evaluation Using 64-Row Multidetector Computed Tomography Angiography) International Multicenter Study. J Am Coll Cardiol 2012;59:379-87.

[10] Douglas PS, Hoffmann U, Lee KL, et al. PROspective Multicenter Imaging Study for Evaluation of chest pain: rationale and design of the PROMISE trial. Am Heart J 2014;167:796-803.e1.

[11] CT coronary angiography in patients with suspected angina due to coronary heart disease (SCOT-HEART): an open-label, parallel-group, multicentre trial. The Lancet;385:2383-91.

[12] Budoff M, Bishop W. Describing the risk demonstrated on cardiac CT imaging: the C-PLUSS approach. Cardiology Today 2015;5(3):23-25

[13] Sarwar A, Shaw LJ, Shapiro MD, et al. Diagnostic and prognostic value of absence of coronary artery calcification. JACC Cardiovasc Imaging 2009;2:675-88.

[14] Malik S, Budoff MJ, Katz R, et al. Impact of subclinical atherosclerosis on cardiovascular disease events in individuals with metabolic syndrome and diabetes the multi-ethnic study of atherosclerosis. Diabetes Care 2011;34:2285-90.

[15] Raggi P, Callister TQ, Cooil B, et al. Identification of patients at increased risk of first unheralded acute myocardial infarction by electron-beam computed tomography. Circulation 2000;101:850-55.

[16] Aslam A, Khokhar US, Chaudhry A, et al. Assessment of isotropic calcium using 0.5-mm reconstructions from 320-row CT data sets identifies more patients with non-zero Agatston score and more subclinical atherosclerosis than standard 3.0-mm coronary artery calcium scan and CT angiography. Journal of cardiovascular computed tomography 2014;8:58-66.

[17] Alliance NVDP. Guidelines for the Management of Absolute Cardiovascular Disease Risk.

[18] Rosen BD, Fernandes V, McClelland RL, et al. Relationship between baseline coronary calcium score and demonstration of coronary artery stenoses during follow-up MESA (Multi-Ethnic Study of Atherosclerosis). JACC Cardiovasc Imaging 2009;2:1175-83.

[19] Raggi P, Cooil B, Callister TQ. Use of electron beam tomography data to develop models for prediction of hard coronary events. Am Heart J;141:375-82.

[20] Bishop W, Heart Rate Preparation. 2012. at http://www.drwarrickbishop.com patient-preparation/.)

Glossary

Acute coronary syndrome/Major Adverse Coronary Event (MACE)
the sudden development of a complete, or near complete, occlusion or blockage, of a coronary artery

complete blockage
myocardial infarction (*myocardial,* the heart; *infarction,* death by lack of blood flow) a complete blockage that causes the death of part of the heart muscle

near complete blockage
or 'unstable angina' puts pressure on the heart and can be the forerunner to a heart attack

Agatston Score
the standardised method of evaluating the coronary arteries for the presence of calcium. Developed by American cardiologist Arthur Agatston, the score uses three millimetre slices through the heart and then a combination of volume and density of the calcium detected to generate a 'score'.

Anatomical
relating to structure

Angina
chest pain experienced in association with reduced flow of blood to the heart. It is not a heart attack but can be an indicator of high risk.

Arteries
the vessels of the body's circulation system that carry the blood away from the heart. The aorta takes the blood from the left ventricle as the blood begins it journey around the body. Coming from the aorta as it leaves the heart are the **right coronary artery** and the **left main coronary artery.**

The left main then divides into two key arteries

the **left anterior descending artery** (LAD) (which provides blood to the anterior surface of the heart, the area nearest the chest wall); generally the most important of the arteries, and

the circumflex artery (which provides blood to the back of the heart, the area nearest the spine), as well as

the right coronary artery (which provides blood to the surface of the heart the area nearest the diaphragm).

Association
connected, joined or related

Asymptomatic
producing or showing no symptoms

Atheroma
build-up of plaque within an artery

Atherosclerotic/atheromatous plaque

the build-up of cholesterol, scavenger cells, scar tissue and calcium in the wall of the artery (referred to as plaque throughout the book). The plaque can be either flow-limiting (and likely to produce symptoms) or non-flow-limiting (produces no symptoms). Also see plaque and plaque burden.

Atrium

a pre-pumping chamber (before the ventricle) on both sides of the heart

Australian absolute cardiovascular disease risk calculator

an approach to predicting risk of cardiovascular disease developed by the National Vascular Disease Prevention Alliance (NVDPA) which is an alliance of four Australian charities: Diabetes Australia, the National Heart Foundation of Australia, Kidney Health Australia and the National Stroke Foundation

Blood

the bodily fluid that conveys oxygen and nutrients to the body and removes carbon dioxide and other wastes. It carries:

platelets

small cellular fragments that are important in the forming of clots when the vascular system is damaged, e.g., they stop a cut from bleeding

red cells

the carriers of the protein, haemoglobin, which transports oxygen around the body. Red cells also remove some of the body's carbon dioxide.

Causations

factors/actions that cause the problem

Cholesterol

a lipid or fat molecule that is used as a component of cell walls and is also a precursor to synthesis of a number of hormones

Computed Tomography (CT)

see electron beam computed tomography

Coronary atheroma burden

term used, in a primary preventative setting, to describe the build-up of plaque within the arteries in a patient who is otherwise well (before the development of disease)

Coronary artery bypass grafting

major surgery that allows a 'bypassing' of the diseased section of the artery by using an alternate vessel, usually from the aorta, to supply blood to the heart

Coronary Artery Calcium (CAC)

the presence of calcium in the arteries (not quantified)
See also Coronary Calcium Score.

Coronary artery disease or heart disease

the process of atherosclerosis or plaque build-up in the artery that leads to a narrowing of the artery and reduced blood flow that produces symptoms (angina, shortness of breath, a heart attack)

Coronary Calcium Score (CCS)

the number, or score, generated when looking to use calcium as a marker of

plaque; the quantification of CAC
See also Agatston Score.

Coronary Computed Tomography Angiogram (CCTA)
the result when contrast (dye) injected into a patient's vein outlines the coronary arteries in exquisite detail, giving information about the location, the quality and nature of the plaque, the degree of stenosis and the size of the vessel affected
Often referred to as a CT coronary angiogram.

C-PLUSS
an acronym to help evaluate and report risk: C (Calcium score), P (calcium score Percentile), L (Low attention plaque), U (Unfavourable positive remodelling), S (Stenosis), S (Site of plaque)

Coronary risk
the possibility of a coronary event such as a heart attack:

low a less than 10 percent chance of a coronary event within 10 years

intermediate between 10 and 20 percent chance of a coronary event within 10 years

high a greater than 20 percent chance of a coronary event within 10 years

CT coronary angiogram
see Coronary Computed Tomography Angiogram (CCTA)

Disease
a symptom or loss of normal function

Distal
situated away from the centre

Echocardiogram (Echo)
a scan of the heart using ultrasound waves to acquire a picture, like a bat uses sonar
It gives information about the valves, the chambers of the heart and pressures within the heart.

Electrocardiogram (ECG)
a trace of the electrical activity through the heart acquired by electrodes
It shows the rhythm of the heart.
Features of the ECG can be used to infer the status of the heart muscle, such as ischaemia seen during a stress test.

Electron Beam Computed Tomography (EBCT)
X-rays are deflected at very high speed using enormous magnets to acquire images that are then reconstructed. This has given rise to the term Computed Tomography (CT).

Evidence-based medicine
the guidelines or recommendations (that help in the management of patients that are put together by specialty groups or organisations) are founded on research in an area
There are different levels of evidence based on the quality and amount of the research available.

Familial hypercholesterolaemia
a generic condition that gives rise to very elevated levels of cholesterol and is associated with a family history of premature coronary artery disease

Fluoroscopy
rapid acquisition x-ray to allow
assessment during movement

Framingham-type risk modelling
using multiple associations with observed
outcomes to predict likelihood of an event
or risk

Heart
a large muscle that pumps blood through
the body

Heart attack
not a medical expression
It is a layman's term referring to a major
heart problem. Most commonly it is a
narrowing of the coronary arteries that
can kill or requires some form of medical
intervention – medication, time in
hospital, balloons or stents, or coronary
artery bypass grafting.

Heart Foundation
a national charity dedicated to fighting
the single biggest killer of Australians,
heart disease
It funds life-saving heart research
and works to improve heart disease
prevention and care for all Australians.

Ischaemic heart disease
reduced blood supply to the heart

Invasive coronary angiogram
direct injection of contrast (dye) into the
coronary arteries by using a thin plastic
catheter (tube) that is passed from the
artery of the leg or from the artery of the
wrist to the origin of the aorta and guided
into the origin of the left main or right

coronary arteries
It gives very precise images of the lumen
or inside of the arteries (the inside of the
artery, not the wall).

Lipid tests
current testing for lipids covers total
cholesterol, triglycerides, high-density
lipoprotein, low-density lipoprotein,
non-high-density lipoprotein and total
cholesterol to HDL ratio

Lipoprotein
the carrier of cholesterol in the blood
(*lipo,* fat)

Lumen
the inside space of the artery, where the
blood flows

Macrophages
scavenger cells, important in the build-
up of plaque

**Major Adverse Coronary Event
(MACE)**
medical term for heart attack (see acute
coronary syndrome)

Myocardium
myo, muscle; *cardium,* being of the
heart, the muscle of the heart

**National Vascular Disease
Prevention Alliance (NVDPA)**
an alliance of four Australian charities:
Diabetes Australia, the National Heart
Foundation of Australia, Kidney Health
Australia and the National Stroke
Foundation

Negative predictive test
the condition is not present

Plaque
the build-up of cholesterol, scavenger cells, scar tissue and calcium in the wall of the artery (referred to as plaque throughout the book)
The plaque can be either flow-limiting (and likely to produce symptoms) or non-flow-limiting (produces no symptoms).

> **unstable plaque** When the fibrous cap of the plaque ruptures, platelets in the blood begin to clump together to form a clot which may completely block the artery.
> If it is a non-flow-limiting plaque, death may occur without any previous warning.

Plaque burden

> **non-calcific/cholesterol dominant/low attenuation plaque (LAP)** the build-up of lipid or fat within the plaque, has a bearing on the stability of the plaque, generally reducing plaque stability
>
> **calcific dominant** the presence of calcium in the plaque greater than the non-calcific component, generally associated with greater plaque stability

Premature coronary disease
suffering a MACE at less than approximately 55 years of age for a male and 60 years of age for a female

Preventative cardiology

> **primary**
> involves treatment of the unknown
> Patients do not display symptoms, yet they may be at high risk because of indicators such as cholesterol levels, high blood pressure, diabetes or smoking. It attempts to prevent the development of coronary disease in a patient who has not suffered an event but indicators suggest could be at risk.
>
> **secondary**
> involves treatment after diagnosis – those strategies that can be put in place because symptoms have been detected or an event, such as a heart attack, has occurred
>
> **risk assessment**
> **population based,** using multiple parameters (for example age, sex, blood pressure) to make an evaluation of an individual's chance of a MACE based on the observed rate of events in a population with the same parameters
>
> **individual based,** imaging the arteries of an individual to make an assessment of the chance of a MACE based on the actual features seen within the individual's arteries
>
> **observational data**
> Databases have been compiled of features and factors found in individuals who have had coronary artery disease. The occurrence of those features and factors then lends weight to their being used as predictors for people before they have an event. This data is collected from a large number of patients. These factors are associations, not necessarily the cause, of the problem.

Proximal
situated nearer to the centre

Radiation
background radiation exposure of a
person over a year through incidental
exposure from things such as rocky
outcrops, electronic devices, atmospheric,
flying in commercial aircraft

Randomised double-blind
control trial
a trial design
The trial takes a population to be studied
and separates the population into two
groups in a random way ('randomised').
One group receives the intervention and
the other group (the 'control' group)
receives **no** intervention.
Neither group knows if it is being given
the true intervention or not (they are
'blinded') and the medical staff who
look after the subjects are not aware of
who is receiving the true intervention or
not (they are 'blind' also). This is called
'double-blind'.

Remodelling
a process in which the vessels change
shape
   positive remodelling
   the vessel enlarges to accommodate
   the atheroma build-up within the
   artery wall

Statins
a family of drugs that lowers cholesterol

Stenosis
narrowing (of the artery)

Stenting
a coronary artery disease intervention
In the intervention, an intravascular
device (balloon) within a wire scaffold
is inserted percutaneously (through the
skin), using similar technique to invasive
coronary angiography, and guided to the
site of a narrowing.
When the balloon is inflated, the artery
is opened and the wire scaffold remains
to keep it open; the scaffold is called
a **stent.** If a wire scaffold is not used
during a ballooning procedure, then it is
called **balloon angioplasty**.

Stress test
a functional test
It tests heart function. It involves
exercising the patient or giving the
patient medication to replicate exercise,
to try to reproduce the symptom under
investigation or unmask lack of blood
flow to the heart.

Stroke
a sudden blockage, or partial blockage, of
a blood vessel supplying the brain
   thrombo-embolic stroke
   when a clot which forms in the carotid
   arteries of the neck breaks off, travels
   to the brain circulation and lodges in
   a vessel, causing lack of blood supply
   beyond that point (*embolic:* carried
   through the blood stream)
   thrombotic stroke
   when a plaque ruptures and a clot
   forms at that site

haemorrhagic stroke
when a ruptured blood vessel in the
brain leads to bleeding into the brain

**atrial fibrillation thrombo-
embolic stroke**
when the chambers at the top of
the heart lose their synchronicity,
contraction of the atria fails, blood
pools within the atrium, a clot forms,
breaks free and lodges in a brain
artery

Troponin
a blood test used as a predictor when a
person presents with chest pain to assess
likelihood of the heart being involved

Veins
the vessels of the body's circulation
system that carry the blood **to** the heart
The blood collects into two major veins,
the superior vena cava and the inferior
vena cava, before draining into the right
atrium and then right ventricle.

Ventricle
the main compression (pumping)
chamber of the heart that pushes the
blood through the body
There is a right and left ventricle.

Acknowledgements

I would like to thank

- » my wife for her tolerance;

- » my other family and friends for their support and understanding;

- » my staff who are always fantastic – we all work together to make a meaningful difference in people's lives;

- » my patients who have engaged in an approach to risk management with belief and focus, with particular acknowledgement to those whose case histories and testimonies are included in the book;

- » my colleagues who have listened to me, encouraged me and tried to understand my perspective, and

- » my colleagues who have not heard me, who have dismissed my ideas and have drawn conclusions before listening; each of you has encouraged me to try to find a voice through this book.

A particular thanks goes to my collaborators, researchers and reviewers without whose help this book would still be a good idea awaiting its time:

» Penny West suffered the first round of typing;

» Alice Saul helped with the early referencing;

» Debra Quartararo helped with the website and front cover;

» John Saul provided valuable feedback and friendship at every stage;

» Kelvin Aldred offered frank patient-specific feedback throughout;

» Alistair Begg provided collegial support and encouragement;

» John Nemarich gave valuable patient feedback;

» Michael McCarthy for GP review and feedback;

» my Dad made edits and suggestions that made it into the book;

» Uncle Rod Miller edited above and beyond the call of duty;

» Jillian Smith brought precision and attention to detail in her editing and proofreading;

» Charles Wooley was good enough to find the time for a low-carb beer and a foreword, in the midst of his very busy schedule;

» Frank Parish provided invaluable radiology expertise;

» Shane Anthony was a master of referencing;

» Karam Kostner, Gerald Watts and Daniel Friedman, colleagues who I hold in the highest regard, were good enough to find precious time in their busy schedules to offer feedback and edits;

» Cathy McAuliffe and I met through the internet. Her help with design has been fantastic and her professionalism without blemish, and

» Penny Edman, my ghost-writer, has been the best. I could not have done it without her. Her focus and enthusiasm have been undaunted, her passion such that I wonder if we are like two proud parents of the pages you have just read.

I am truly grateful for all the help and support.

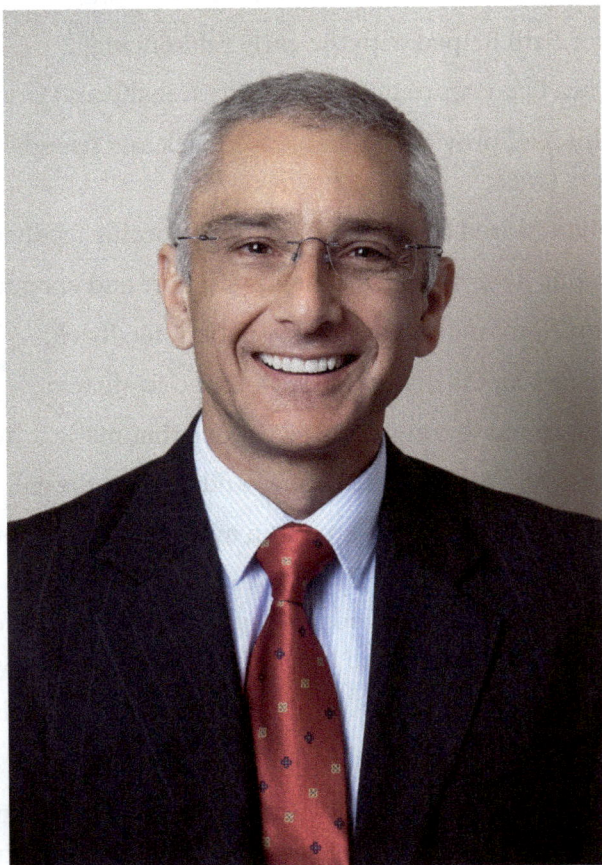
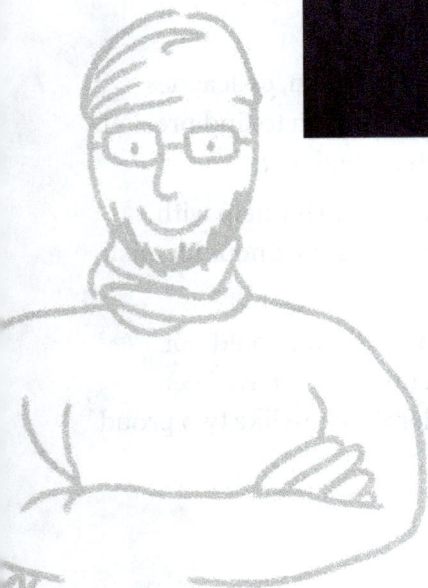

About the author

Warrick Bishop is a practising cardiologist with an interest in cardiovascular disease prevention and a special interest in cardiac CT imaging, lipid management and eating guidelines.

He graduated from the University of Tasmania, School of Medicine, in 1988. He worked in the Northern Territory and subsequently commenced his specialist training in Adelaide, South Australia. He completed his advanced training in cardiology in Hobart, Tasmania, becoming a fellow of the Royal Australian College of Physicians in 1997.

He has worked predominately in private practice, combined with public sessions. In 2009 Warrick undertook training in CT Cardiac Coronary Angiography, being the first cardiologist in Tasmania with this specialist recognition. This area of imaging fits well with his interest in preventative cardiology. He holds level B certification with the Australian Joint Committee for CCTA and is a member of the Society of Cardiac Computed Tomography.

Warrick is also a member of the Australian Atherosclerosis Society and a participant on the panel of 'interested parties' developing a model of care and national registry for familial hypercholesterolaemia. He has also developed a particular interest in diabetic-related risk of coronary artery disease, specifically related to eating guidelines and lipid profiles.

Warrick is an accredited examiner for the Royal Australian College of Physicians and is regularly involved with teaching medical students and junior doctors. He has worked with Hobart's Menzies Institute for Medical Research on projects in an affiliate capacity and is recognised by the Medical School of the University of Tasmania with academic status.

For more than a year, Warrick has been a member of the Clinical Issues Committee of the Australian Heart Foundation, providing input into issues of significance for the management of heart patients.

In his free time, Warrick enjoys travel and music with his wife, and he surfs and plays guitar with his children.

www.ingramcontent.com/pod-product-compliance
Lightning Source LLC
Chambersburg PA
CBHW072059020426
42334CB00017B/1572

* 9 7 8 0 6 4 6 9 6 2 6 7 2 *